KRIYA YOGA: INSIGHTS ALONG THE PATH

by

Marshall Govindan and Jan Ahlund

Babaji's Kriya Yoga and Publications, Inc.

St. Etienne de Bolton, Quebec, Canada

Kriya Yoga: Insights along the path
by Marshall Govindan and Jan Ahlund

First published in April 2008 by
Babaji's Kriya Yoga and Publications, Inc.
196 Mountain Road, P.O. Box 90,
Eastman, Quebec, Canada J0E 1P0
Telephone: 450-297-0258; 1-888-252-9642; fax: 450-297-3957
· www.babajiskriyayoga.net · email: info@babajiskriyayoga.net

Cover design and graphic layout: Sonia Giguere

Printed and bound in Canada. 100% printed on recycled paper

Government of Québec – Tax credit for book publishing- Administered by SODEC.

Care has been taken to trace the ownership of any copyright material contained in this text.

Library and Archives Canada Cataloguing in Publication

Govindan, Marshall
    Kriya Yoga: insights along the path / Marshall Govindan and Jan "Durga" Ahlund

ISBN 978-1-895383-49-2

    1. Yoga, Kriya. I. Ahlund, Jan Suzanne II. Title.

BL1238.56.K74G693 2008   294.5'436   C2008-901944-X

CONTENTS

PREFACE

My wife, Jan "Durga" Ahlund and I have recognized for many years the need for a book that would explain to both those interested in learning Kriya Yoga and those already embarked on its path, why they should practice it, what are the difficulties, and how to overcome them. We believe that this book will help prepare everyone for the challenges and opportunities that Kriya Yoga provides. Every one of us faces the resistance of our human nature, ignorance as to our true identity, and karma, the consequences of years of conditioning by our thoughts, words and actions. By cultivating aspiration for the Divine, rejecting egoism and its manifestations, and surrendering to our higher Self, pure Witness consciousness, we can overcome this resistance, our karma and the many obstacles on the path. But, to do so, we need much support and insight along the way.

Marshall Govindan and Jan Ahlund
March 12, 2008
St Etienne de Bolton, Quebec, Canada

PART 1

The Dilemma of human existence: Finding lasting happiness in things which do not last

1. Why Do We Practice Yoga?

One of the most important debates every student must win is one with their own mind over the doubt: "Why do I practice Yoga?" Until you are convinced of the value of Yoga relative to everything else in your life, your practice will not have the priority needed to escape your suffering. Your mind will create endless doubts and distractions until you begin to establish yourself in a perspective that transcends it. Read carefully, and absorb the implications of what is the most important debate of your life.

A change in perspective:

In one form or another we are all suffering. Individually and collectively. We may try to deny it, or avoid it, but it is pervasive. Our suffering takes so many forms: physical pain; emotional grief, fear, anger, envy, expectations regarding others, mental worry; depression. We seek to escape it through alcohol, drugs, television, eating, exercise, innumerable forms of distraction, work, therapy, and religion. Rarely do we take time to understand the root cause of our suffering, or why we cause so much suffering to one another. We rarely remember that everything in life is impermanent. Everything we experience changes: our physical circumstances, our emotional and mental state, our physical condition, our relationships, and our financial situation. And yet we often react with surprise, anger, disappointment, even shock when loved ones die, or things break, or we lose our job, or experience an accident or a betrayal. We foolishly expect to find lasting happiness in things which do not last!

Wisdom is to know the source of suffering, the source of joy, and to distinguish what is permanent from what is impermanent. The wise tell us that it is the confusion of our true Self with that of the body-mind-personality, which is at the root of suffering. They tell us that when we identify with our soul, standing firmly in the perspective of an inner Witness, we can know profound joy, instantly and effortlessly.

Who is it that suffers? There may be physical pain, turbulent emotions, troubling thoughts. But they come and go. And when they are gone, who we truly are remains. You are that which always is, throughout the passing spectacle of physical sensations, emotions and thoughts. You cannot be anything that comes and goes. You can only be that which always is and never changes. Take a few deep breaths now, and ask yourself: "What part of me never changes?" Thoughts change. Emotions change. The body's sensations change. What is left? Do not even put a label on it. Just notice "it." "It" is formless, timeless, unchanging. It is the one constant throughout all of the experiences of your life. It was present when you were five years old, seventeen years old, thirty years old, and it will be present in the last years, and moments of your life. It is like the thread upon which the string of pearls is strung. We rarely notice it, yet it is our true Self, your soul. Wisdom is to establish oneself in the perspective of this one constant, 24/7.

Due to the fact that your mind is engaged in reading this article, trying to understand the point I am making, thoughts are arising. But can you take a step back and change your perspective, becoming a Witness to whatever thoughts, feelings, sensations arise as you continue to read this article? If you can, you will be enjoying the perspective of your soul, which is pure consciousness. However, unlike everything else, "it" cannot be experienced, because it is not an object. It is the subject. Everything else is object. So, realizing "Who" you are is not about having a new experience. There is nothing "special" to experience. You are not going to become "special" either. Being "special" implies being apart from everything else. Who you are is that which is behind every "thing," and therefore non-separate.

"It" cannot be understood either. Understanding implies thoughts about an object of observation or consideration. But "it" is beyond all thoughts. It is simply love.

You are not your thoughts. Most of them are not even yours to begin with. You have thoughts; they come and they go. But you remain. Most of the thoughts are generated by others, float around in the mental atmosphere and then they enter your field of mental consciousness, where you add a little local color, a little personal twist, and then you express it with "I think," or "I'm discouraged," "I must do this," or "I am angry or afraid" or whatever.

So, the wise are those who can change perspective, and remain in a state of realization wherein they identify not with thoughts, emotions and sensations of the body-mind, but with the Witness perspective of the soul. The Witness perspective of the soul is wide-giving love.

Egoism

Why do we ordinarily identify our self with our sensations and emotions? In the span of one day we are apt to confuse "who we are" with several, often conflicting, sensations and emotions. "I am happy," I think upon awakening. The day is sunny and the drive to work is easy and indeed, "I am unflappable." After a cup of coffee and two difficult phone calls, "I am angry and stressed." Later in the day, "I am envious or jealous" due to the accomplishments and praise given by a co-worker. By the end of one day, and after a long stressful drive home, "I" might have identified myself as being happy, calm, bored, jealous, envious, unsettled, furious. "I" might even find "I hate" a person who "I adored" earlier in the day or visa versa. "I" cannot be all these changing emotions and sensations.

So which of these describe "who you are?" "You" are not any of these things.

If I ask you who you are, you may tell me your name, and what you do for a living; perhaps your marital status and to whom you are related to, like the "mother/father of three children." You may tell me where you are from, what you like, what you do not like; where you work, your politics, your religion. If we have more time you begin to tell me stories about yourself and what you believe. However, if I meet you a year later, any of these may have changed, you may have lost your job, gotten divorced, changed your political and religious affiliations and changed what you like and do not like about the world. And now you have new stories to tell me. So, who are you? Really? You cannot be any of the above, because they are all temporary. You can only be that which never changes. Because if it changes; it no longer is.

We are so confused about our identity. We say or think "I" a thousand plus times a day! But who is this "I"? The word for "I" in Greek is "ego." Ego may be defined as the habit of identifying with the body, mind, and emotions. Whenever we do or think or feel something repeatedly, a habit forms. The interior lobes of the brain program our habits to facilitate our responses to external stimuli, coming through the five senses. We have thousands of habits, which are unique to each individual. The way we walk, talk, eat, drive a car, treat others, the things we like and don't like, all these are based upon habits. Taken together, their sum adds up to what is referred to as our *karma*: the consequences of our past thoughts, words and actions. The most significant habit that we each have is the habit of identifying with our thoughts, emotions and sensations. We say or think: "I think" or "I feel" or "I am suffering" or "I am angry." However, truly, we are not anything of these experiences. It is correct to say: "Here's a thought about that" or "my body is tired," or "I am feeling upset about this or that." That is, anything we experience is an object; it is not the subject. Who I truly am, pure Witness consciousness, is the subject. So egoism is really a case of mistaken identity. Like an actor, we pretend that we are someone who we are not, forgetting our true identity.

The Consequences of Egoism

The most important consequence of egoism is suffering. Suffering depends upon how you react to what happens. It is therefore distinct from pain. For instance, pain may occur when you trip and fall and bruise your body. Suffering involves the emotions like anger, embarrassment and regret that follow. Due to egoism, you identify with such emotions, swear and lose your sense of equanimity and humor. Suffering throws you off balance. The ego can be thrown off balance. Who you truly are cannot. Who you truly are, maintains a sense of equanimity. It is therefore important to be vigilant, and notice the manifestations of the ego, before it unbalances and sweeps you away into negative feelings. These include:

1. Desire: imagining or fantasizing the pleasure to be derived from some object or circumstance, or feeling aversion towards something,

which we believe will cause us some pain or discomfort. They are fleeting, but prevent us from enjoying the present moment. Desire is a trap, for any desire will convince us that we would be "better off" if only we could satisfy that desire. It burns until it is satisfied; then there is a temporary suspension of the desire, until, the next desire arises, usually immediately afterwards. Desires are endless. The next time you feel desire for something, ask yourself "Who desires?" Immediately you will turn toward your true self, and see things from its true perspective, that of the Witness. In truth, there is no one who desires; desires come, and then they go away. When you are satisfying a desire, again, watch yourself enjoying it. Cultivate the perspective of a detached loving observer. One who loves, desires nothing.

2. Anger. These include all of those strong passionate feelings held towards something or someone, even oneself, when desires are frustrated. Anger itself is habit-forming. It must be rejected or re-directed. Anger always negatively affects the one who owns it most. The wise do not hold on to anger. Anger can always be re-directed into positive action to help correct a mistake. One who loves cannot hold onto anger.

3. Greed: involves wanting more for yourself, rather than wanting the best for others. Greed is a practice of being self-centered with regard to everything; wanting the lion's share of everything whether it is financial wealth, food, sensual gratification, emotional gratification or spiritual gratification. One, who loves truly, is not greedy.

4. Pride: this is a highly exaggerated opinion of oneself, frequently resulting in contempt for and ill treatment of others. One feels oneself to be somehow superior. It may manifest when one identifies with one's personal accomplishments, or with the accomplishments of a religion, a sports team, one's race, nationality, or whenever there is a thought of "me" or "us" versus "them." Pride hides the realization of our true Self and makes us unable to see the underlying unity of everyone. Pride confines love.

5. Envy, malice and jealousy: the bitterness experienced on seeing others being happy or having something that one does not have. It also obscures the true inner source of joy. Bitterness restricts love so that one is not able to experience it even for oneself.

The wise see these manifestations of the ego as opportunities for self purification: letting go of what one is not, so that one can enjoy the inner source of well being and love.

Working on oneself

The ordinary human being swings on a pendulum between seeking pleasure and avoiding pain. However, both of these involve suffering. Suffering follows even when one obtains what one desires, out of the fear of losing it. The wise, however, find a middle path and cultivate equal-mindedness. Equal-mindedness is contentment and equanimity towards what comes or does not come. It is the litmus test of true spirituality. When asked to describe his state of enlightenment, the great sage, Ramana Maharshi replied: "Now nothing can disturb me anymore." From the perspective of our soul, if it costs one's peace of mind, it costs too much! However, because the mind is addicted to seeking pleasure and avoiding pain, it rarely finds that state of balance. The wise cultivate this balance in thought, word and deed. Everything in the life of the wise becomes an opportunity to cultivate equanimity and love. This does not mean that pain or discomfort or bad karmic consequences cease to intrude into one's life; it does mean that one does not react, but rather responds consciously, cultivating presence, awareness and love. This provides the optimum situation in which inspiration may come and resolve difficulties. It also helps to prevent the needless loss of energy expended in worry, anger, and grief, when things do not go according to plan!

Our true Self is seated beyond the senses that take in, and react to what is happening around us; it is beyond the conditioning of the mind and the intellect, which interprets what is being seen, heard, tasted, touched and felt. Our true being is blessed, seated secretly in limitless, illuminated love and bliss. With this understanding we can transcend the ordinary human perspective of the ego, and access the perspective of our soul, which is one of peace and unconditional love.

Those who have reached the pinnacle of human perfection, the Yoga Siddhas, or perfected ones, did so because of a long process of ego purification. All genuine spiritual traditions emphasize this process. Jesus said: "Listen to me, all of you, and try to understand! It's not what goes into a person from the outside that can defile; rather it's what comes out of the person that defiles." (Mark 7.14-15 with parallels in Matthew 15.10-1 and Thomas 14.5) What comes out of the person is a manifestation of the ego, as described above. How to purify oneself? The inner purity which Jesus is emphasizing here, begins with discrimination against thoughts, words and actions that defile: judgment, greed, lust, anger, hatred and desire. All of these cause suffering for others and for the person harboring them. Words and actions are preceded by thoughts, so one must develop awareness of the negative mental tendencies and detach from then as soon as they begin to manifest within.

The practice of meditation helps one to develop the presence and awareness necessary to do this. But one cannot expect that merely going deep into meditation is going to miraculously transform one's everyday behavior. One must learn to bring the detached perspective of the soul into the challenging moments of everyday life. This process can be summarized in two acts of spiritual discipline, which define Classical Yoga: "Yoga is remembering Who AM I, and letting go of what I am not." Like the two wings of a bird they lift one to the perspective of a realizing a heaven on earth. For, where is God not? Only where we are not truly present. It also requires a direct approach to negative thoughts and tendencies. Patanjali tells us in Yoga-sutra II.33: "When bound by negative thoughts, their opposites should be cultivated." This may be done, for example, by blessing others, rather than judging them, loving them rather than hating them, repeating affirmations, auto-suggestions, visualization exercises and prayer.

Too often we sink into worry and depression when invaded by negative thoughts. Worry and depression is meditating on what we do not want! The wise, realizing that all manifestations begin in the mind, cultivate the best of thoughts and feelings through meditation in daily life. This entails cultivating a continuous stream of awareness with regards to all happenings. Awareness occurs when part of one's consciousness stands back and watches what the rest of the consciousness is engaged in. It does not think; it watches thoughts coming and going. It does not do anything; it watches things happening. It does not feel. The Witness is equal-minded loving compassion, which watches emotions arising and subsiding in the vital part of ones body. With a little practice, it becomes the foundational perspective of one's life, ensuring a state that is quite the opposite of "egoism and suffering." Being present, one is automatically aware, and when one is aware, bliss arises. So "presence and love" replace "egoism and suffering." This is the promise of those who have successfully scaled the Mt. Everest of ordinary human nature, and arrived at the peak of Self-realization.

Egoism is a principle of nature by which consciousness becomes contracted around objects of experience. Every living creature experiences this contraction of consciousness primarily within the range of its senses. The consciousness of the ordinary person, for example, is absorbed in physical sensations during childhood. As one matures, one becomes absorbed in mental and emotional movements: fantasies, fear and desires. Later, one gets caught up in thoughts: memories, ideas and problems. This contraction of consciousness around objects of experience, be they physical, emotional, mental or intellectual, is due to egoism. It is not a personal defect. It is part of nature's design, which relates to the fundamental existential question: why did the One become many? And how can one return to the state of oneness?

According to the sages, beyond this ephemeral world of objective nature, there is a higher "causal plane" from which everything originates. Suffering motivates everyone to go beyond the limited perspective of the ego, but with more or less wisdom. The unwise do so through distraction. The wise, perceiving the Reality beyond the surface, expand their consciousness through spiritual disciplines and secure unconditional, unchallenged love in their hearts in order to purifying the ego based consciousness, and as a result, realize ever new joy in a state of Self realization.

Practical means to uncover egoism:

1. Do something for others every day, without expecting anything in return as selfless service. This can involve any activity, even in your work if done in a spirit of detached awareness, while seeing the Divine in others.

2. Meditate on love: that which is behind the surface movements of the body, mind and emotions.

3. Cultivate detachment. This feeling of letting go is the opposite of "attachment," which we often confuse with love. See yourself on the riverbank of thoughts and experiences, watching them flow by. Avoid slipping down into the river of thoughts and being carried away by them.

4. Cultivate calmness. Be calmly active: when you respond to the world, respond calmly and with care. Actively work to remain calm, re-

gardless of what is happening around you. Calmness is the window of our soul. By cultivating it, we see the Presence of Love everywhere.

5. "Self study": keep a journal in which you record your experiences. Notice the habits of your mind. Study sacred, spiritual texts which remind you of your higher, true Self.

6. Before speaking, reflect, and speak only what is true, necessary, helpful and uplifting.

7. Stretch your body and watch your breathing. Take up a discipline of body mind spirit exercises, which help to manage stress, relax you deeply and increase energy. By managing our stress and relaxing deeply, we can avoid the ego's tendency to get "caught up" in the dramas of our lives.

8. The food you eat can affect your thoughts. Eat consciously and don't allow unconscious thoughts to predominate in your mind. Bad food habits can perpetuate fear, depression, anger or unhappiness in your life. Eating poorly or too much will deplete your energy level. When you do not feel energetic you will be less able to let go of identification with your body.

9. Cultivate the opposite of negative thoughts and feelings through affirmations and auto-suggestions.

10. Enjoy your daily life by living it consciously. Make each day as beautiful as possible. Opportunities arise in the moment. Be conscious of each moment. Walk consciously really seeing what is in front of you.

The cultivation of practices like these can help to raise your consciousness above the limited perspective of "me," "myself," and "I." Make a conscious effort to move beyond the ego and become "a light unto oneself." Others will find joy in your presence.

2. Karma: Cause or Consequence?

The term "karma" brings to mind notions of law and justice, reward and punishment, as well as judgment and fate. In the Christian and Judaic context it also seems to include the concept of sin and punishment. As such, it is not something we care to dwell upon; but rather dread. Because it is related to such difficult concepts, we generally prefer to avoid thinking about it; too often our attitude is "I don't understand it," or "it is difficult to understand." But whether we understand it or not, we are all subject to this law of Nature.

If we do think about "karma" it raises so many unanswered questions, including:

1. Why do we create karma?

2. What types of karma are there?

3. Why do bad things happen to good people?

4. Is my life determined by fate or by my free will?

5. What can I do to overcome bad karma?

6. What is grace? What does it have to do with karma? How to obtain it?

7. How can Kriya Yoga neutralize karma?

Before attempting to answer these questions, however, let us attempt to define karma, and then to understand its origins.

Karma defined: A simple definition is that karma is a law or principle of nature, which requires that every action, word or thought has an effect or consequence; or that every action has a reaction. When often repeated, such thoughts, words and actions also have a cumulative effect, which manifests as subconscious habits, or tendencies. So karma is cause and consequence.

What is the origin of the concept of karma?

Karma is not a concept limited to Eastern philosophy or religions. It is referred to in so many words in the Judaic-Christian traditions in reference to "sin," "judgment," and "salvation." For example, "As you sow, so shall you reap." It is referred to in the western scientific literature with reference to "cause and effect." It is at the heart of every person's sense of "justice" and "fairness." Even the term "law," is based upon notions of karma.

References to notions of karma are found in the oldest religion of the world, known as the Vedic religion, whose origins go back to nearly 10,000 B.C. It was essentially a monistic religion, but recognized various "gods" which represented the powers of the one Lord, Brahman. It was, and is to this day, a religion that uses sacrificial offerings, particularly into a sacred fire, as a means of pleasing the gods and of acquiring merit. The notions underlying karma, that is, giving and receiving, merit and demerit, righteous versus unrighteous conduct, undoubtedly grew out of these religions practices.   It was believed the Vedic gods sometimes needed to be appeased, particularly after unmeritorious or unrighteous actions by human folk and their leaders.   In the Old Testament we find such expressions as "An eye for an eye, and a tooth for a tooth," which also reflects an appreciation for notions of karma.

Question number 1: Why do we create karma?

In Yoga-Sutra II.12, Patanjali refers to types of karma: "The reservoir of karma rooted in the afflictions is experienced in seen (present) and unseen (future) existence."

He is referring to several important concepts, and their relationship to karma. First, he is referring to a "reservoir" or "womb" of karma or "action deposits" that each soul carries with it from life to life. Thoughts, words, actions, when often repeated, form habits, and these habits form tendencies that determine how we react to similar situations in the future. Like seeds, these tendencies, or *samskaras* wait for an opportunity to sprout, under the right conditions, in our present life, or in a future incarnation. Even without believing in reincarnation, one can understand the influence of one's genes.

Secondly, he is referring to the afflictions: five causes of suffering. Previously he defined these as (1) ignorance as to our true identity, as soul, ignorance as to what is permanent, and what brings joy versus what brings suffering (2) egoism, the habit of identifying with the body-mind and its thoughts and feelings, (3) attachment, clinging to pleasure, (4) aversion, clinging to suffering, and (5) clinging to life. The five afflictions are the motivators for creating karma.

For example, when we feel or say, "I want," "I need" or "I am afraid," we are expressing one or more of these afflictions. Realization of "Who am I?" allows us to overcome the first affliction, and as a result, sets the stage for resolving the others. The body may be tired. There may be thoughts of desire, or feelings of anger, but "I" am not the fatigue, the desire, nor the anger. "I am" the one who witnesses them, says the Self-realized. The "witness" is not doing anything; the "witness" is watching things get done. The "witness" is not thinking; the "witness" is watching the thoughts come and go. Patanjali advises us, that by practicing meditation with emphasis on detachment, we develop this perspective of being the Witness, pure consciousness. As a result we may begin to overcome these afflictions. But only by returning to the source of our being, in a state of Self-realization can one uproot these sources of suffering.

Question number 2: What types of karma are there? Is there Good Karma? Bad Karma?

In the above verse, Patanjali is also referring to the present and future existences. Karma is of three types:

1. fate, those presently being expressed and exhausted through this birth;

2. new karmas being created during this birth;

3. those waiting to be fulfilled in future births;

The *karmas* wait for an opportunity to come to the surface and to express themselves through the above-mentioned causes of affliction. For example, a soul with a strong need to express itself through music, may take birth into a family where music is highly valued and cultivated as an art. One strong *karma* may call for a particular birth and body to express itself, and other closely related karmas will also be expressed or exhausted through it.

We need to understand that much, but not all of our life is the result of our karmic destiny. We have our own karmic "map" and "bank balance" that we are born with, but we continue to add to it, positively or negatively. We also need to understand that each person has his own *karma* and acts according to it. We wonder why someone acts a certain way, or lives a certain way. He is wondering the same about us. Each of us is programmed with certain karmic tendencies. Our opinions of what is good or great come from what we were taught and how well we have learned our lessons. The circumstances of our life occur because of our *karma*. But this does not mean that everything in our life is predetermined. We have free will as to how we will deal with these circumstances and events in life, positively or negatively. But we must be aware of both our tendencies to react in a habitual way, and our freedom to act consciously. If we choose to react to life's challenges negatively, for example, in creating suffering for others, the reactions return to us in more intense or terrible forms. Dealing with circumstances patiently, creating happiness for others, neutralizes the karmic consequences gradually.

To identify the major lines of one's karma the following exercise is suggested: Answer the following questions: What have been your life's major desires? Your major fears? What have you been most attached to? What things have caused you the most suffering? What have been your life's major events? Turning points? Lessons?

Then reflect on this statement: To break free of *karma* we must realize what is our purpose in this life.

Good and Bad karma?

In Yoga-Sutra II.14, Patanjali tells us: "Because of virtuous and non-virtuous karma, there are [corresponding] pleasurable and painful consequences."

If we bring happiness to others we gain pleasure; if we bring suffering to others we will reap pain for ourselves. If we allow true happiness for ourselves, we automatically make others who are near us happier -- whether or not they know that initially. Our subconscious habits, largely determine our actions. Therefore, the quality of our birth, lifespan, and life experience is determined by the seeds we sow in our subconscious. To avoid reinforcing negative habits, such as judging others, getting angry, or hurting others with our words, we should first listen to and reflect on our innermost guidance, and avoid egoistic reactions. To reinforce positive habits we should cultivate thoughts, words and deeds, which will be uplifting to ourselves, and to others. Recognize and attend to the promptings of conscience before reacting, and the feelings of guilt which indicate where we have erred. Ask yourself: "How can I say this without harming this person?" "Does my statement imply a judgment about them?" "How will this person feel if I do or say this?"

To reinforce the distinction between good and bad karma, the following exercise is suggested:

When you have consciously made an effort to say or do something you knew would bring joy to others; How did you feel as a result?

When you have avoided saying or doing something you knew would harm others? How did you feel? When you failed to avoid them? How did you feel afterwards? When you have said something that you knew would be harmful? How did you feel?

Consider doing this exercise regularly, before going to bed at night, upon reflection of the day's events.

Question number 3: Why do bad things happen to good people?

When accidents, acts of aggression, natural disasters, or unexpected losses occur, causing suffering or death to persons who appear to be completely innocent, or who have lived virtuous lives, we may well wonder "Why do bad things happen to good people?" The cause may be either of the first two types cited above: (1) fate, those karmas brought into this life and presently being expressed and exhausted through this birth or (2) the consequences of acts performed in this life. A good person in this life generally does not commit acts that would result in terrible consequences. When the bad things are really terrible, usually it is the former: inescapable fate, the consequence of past life actions. Small errors of judgment or mistakes in words or actions do, of course, bring consequences, often immediately. But the above question is usually in response to tragic events that occur to the innocent. Their previous lives' karma is bearing consequences in this life not only for themselves, but for their loved ones too. For example, when a young girl is raped, how is the father of the young girl affected? Is there a connection between his suffering and his own fate? The answer is both personal and complex. The adage "the sins of the father are visited upon the sons" may apply here as well. We share karma with our loved ones, not only genetically, but in the lessons that we teach one another, especially about the meaning of love. We suffer, for example when we confuse love with attachment. Love is giving. Attachment is giving with expectation and brings disappointment and pain when the expectation is not fulfilled. Our suffering becomes our greatest teacher. By going into the suffering deeply and through it ultimately, we become liberated from it.

Some choose to believe in predestination, and discount the power to act consciously.

A suggested practice to overcome fears of bad things happening is to make a list of things you worry about. Afterwards, ask yourself "why"? Record what comes up for you. Then contemplate on the following: "Who worries?" and "Worry is meditation on what you don't want."

Question number 4: Is my life determined by destiny, fate or by my free will?

While destiny, fate and karma are related, they are not equivalent. Destiny is those events that occur despite all of one's efforts to bring about an alternative result. It is karma, the consequences of a previous incarnation's actions being realized in the present life. Fate is the consequence of a lack of will to change or overcome one's habits. Fate is the result of the balance between the good and bad karma, the positive and the negative habits one has cultivated.

Karma as we have seen earlier is of several types and includes a play between good and bad karma. One may mitigate bad karma, which has caused suffering to others by good karma, such as charitable acts, which brings joy to others. This mitigation may occur in the present life, for example, in the case of a former criminal whose subsequent acts of kindness touches others and earns their love and respect. Or someone who works so hard, that despite a lack of education or other advantages, succeeds in their career. Knowing that all thoughts, words and actions bear consequences, the wise therefore avoid evil and seek only the good. The wise are attentive to opportunities "to do good." In this way they accumulate a great positive balance of merit, which may offset or at least weaken the effects of evil acts. They speak only what is necessary and edifying for others. They recognize the great opportunities that exist in acts of charity and compassion. By acting selflessly they also purify themselves of egoism. The deluded on the other hand, act from egoism, and seek advantage for themselves over others. In so doing they cause pain to others, and inevitable karmic consequences for themselves, either in the present or future incarnations. They also strengthen their own egoism, and sink further into delusion.

Destiny is unavoidable karma, no matter how great is one's balance of positive karma. Whether it brings difficulty or pleasure, the way we respond to it is with equanimity, remembering: "this too shall pass." The wise realize that destiny provides to them another opportunity to "let go" of attachments, to remain eqanimous, and to center themselves in the awareness of their underlying being, consciousness and bliss.

Free will is a delusion as long as one is a slave to the ego's fears and desires. Free will can be exercised only when one is aware and unattached to desires, and the dualities of life. By cultivating detachment one sees beyond liking and disliking, success and failure, loss and gain, pleasure and pain, to the Truth of things. Abiding in the awareness of the Truth, one can act "freely," no longer a slave to fear or desire. One can act powerfully as a loving instrument of the Divine. "Not my will but thy will be done," becomes the mantra of those whose will has become freed from egoistic, karmic and deluded tendencies. Otherwise, "free will" is a delusion, merely a servant of egoistic desires and preferences. "I prefer to have…" or "I prefer to do…" says the ego. "It does not matter…" and "I am love" says the soul. Patanjali referred to Kriya Yoga as a remedy for ignorance and egoism: Kriya means "action with awareness," and its systematic practice enables one to bring awareness into all actions, in all five dimensions. It is a powerful antidote to karma: "action with reaction."

Over reliance upon predestination makes one a slave to one's karma, through fear and "self-fulfilling prophecy." One tends to attract what one thinks about. The right use of will coupled with reflective insight and yogic discipline is generally a better use of one's energy and intelligence. One learns to master each situation as it comes. A yogi seeks to surrender to what may come, to purify himself of desires, preferences and fears, and so become a perfect instrument for the Lord. "Not my will but Thy will be done," becomes one's motto, and allows one to ultimately move beyond the feeling of separation from the Divine.

Here are some suggested practices to develop equanimity, "free will" and to mitigate the effects of fate:

1. Repeat these affirmations "Not my will, but thy will be done." Or "May Your Will be done, and not mine," and "As you will, as you will."

2. When the unexpected occurs, before reacting, pause, and reflect. Let go of the emotional reaction.

3. Look for opportunities to bring joy to others. Increase your merit of good karma. Avoid words, thoughts and actions that may bring suffering to others.

Question 5: What can I do to overcome bad karma?

Thoughts lead to words, which lead to actions, which lead to karmic reactions. But good karma can weaken or even neutralize the effects of bad karma. For example, you may harbor many judgmental thoughts about a friend, and one day, your judgment slips out as a verbal remark in their presence and you offend your friend. Realizing your mistake, you later make sincere amends, and so do not lose that person as a friend. Or, you develop the habit of getting very angry when things do not go as you expect. After a period of soul searching, you begin to restrain your temper. But the habit of expressing your anger is so deeply rooted, that you find it difficult to avoid. You may confess, and feel remorse, but you continue to be swept along by the force of your temperament, the karmic tendency you have cultivated. How can one stop it?

Patanjali recommends direct action: "When bound by negative thoughts, their opposite, (i.e., positive) should be cultivated." By negative thoughts, he is referring to all those that lead to difficulties in our human relationships and personal discontent, unconscious behavior and confusion. These include desire, fear, greed, lust, deceit, lying, exaggeration, and any thought, word or deed that may harm others. For example, if you feel resentment towards someone, you can develop thoughts of forgiveness. Similarly, if there is fear, you should cultivate thoughts of courage and confidence. To counter deep-seated karmic tendencies or habits requires regular and diligent practice of such methods as affirmation, and auto-suggestion. The subconscious mind continues to operate according to suggestions programmed into it since early childhood, even when they have caused harm or suffering. Such suggestions come to us from our parents, teachers, friends, the mass media and the cultural symbols and values that permeate our world. Rather than just suppressing unwholesome thoughts and emotions, which leads to neuroses, each person must learn to skillfully counter them.

One can counter that which is unhealthy, by identifying and categorizing habitual negative thinking. Take a thought such as "anger" and compose an affirmation to counter it. An affirmation is a statement in the present tense, and first person, which expresses a positive change in one's life. For example, for anger, it might be something like: "When the unexpected occurs, I enjoy remaining as a calm witness, knowing that this too shall pass." Repeat your affirmation with a positive emotion, three to five times, slowly and with concentration whenever you are in a relaxed state, at least three times per day, for 21 days. You can, for example, affirm before going to sleep at night, after relaxing in your bed, at the end of a meditation or during the relaxation period at the end of a session of yoga practice.

Question number 6: What is grace? What does it have to do with karma?

The concept of grace is found throughout the teachings of most world religions. It reflects the widespread recognition that our prayers are answered by a source of benevolence, independent of whether we are deserving, or not. With karma, we get what we deserve. With grace we receive what is uplifting and edifying to our soul, in response to its call. Just as every action, word or thought has by the law of karma a necessary consequence or reaction, there is a higher law that whereby the sincere call of our soul brings a response from the Lord in the form of grace. This grace can lessen our karma.

While it is beyond the scope of this article to make a case for the existence of a Supreme being, it is pertinent to mention that since we are speaking of "karma," the law of cause and consequence, one can infer that there must be an ultimate cause to every lesser cause. That is, a source for all causes as well as all knowledge, which is deemed the Creator. Many questions arise when one begins to reflect upon the relationship between the Creator or the Lord, and karma. For example, to what extent is the Creator directly involved in the karmas of individual souls? Patanjali tells us "The Lord is the special Self, untouched by any afflictions, actions, fruits of actions (ie. Karma) or by any inner impressions of desires." - Yoga-sutras, I.24. Jesus echoed this when he said: "The Kingdom of God is not coming with signs to be observed, nor will they say, 'Look, here it is!' or 'there!' for behold, the kingdom of God is in the midst of you." (Luke 17.21)   Patanjali goes on to say that "Unconditioned by time, he is the teacher of even the most ancient teachers." Yoga-sutra I.25 This indicates that while the Lord is not affected by karmas and desires, he does not ignore our human condition. He is our ultimate teacher, and he teaches us through karma. Through the law of karma he has created a kind of school for the education of our souls. For what purpose? If the purpose of knowledge is to alleviate human suffering, that knowledge, which eliminates suffering completely, must be the greatest of all knowledge.

The ancient spiritual texts of India speak of the five acts of the Lord: Creation, Preservation, Destruction, Obscuration and Grace. The purpose of the above-mentioned five acts of the Lord is to help the souls get rid of their impurities, which prevent them from seeing the Lord. As Jesus said: "Blessed are the pure in heart, for they will see God." (Matthew 5.8) The five acts are not for His amusement, but because of the Lord's love for the souls. So, the Lord gives souls a body to work out their karma; he supports and preserves them for awhile so that they can experience the results of their actions, and so learn wisdom from them; he gives them rest through destruction of the body; he gives obscuration to veil their true nature as consciousness and eventually bliss, resulting from equanimity with regards to karma; finally he gives them release from the bondage of delusion of separation for the Lord. Thus all of His acts are expressions of His Grace. By them, he ultimately draws us near to Him.

When one seeks lasting happiness in things that do not last, there is bound to be suffering. Everything is temporary: possessions, relationships, circumstances, status, opinions, emotions and thoughts. Even when we fulfill desires there will always be more desires, as well as the desire or even fear not to lose what we have, hence more suffering. Therefore, only that which is permanent and infinite could be the source of lasting happiness. Wisdom is to know the difference between the permanent and the impermanent, and consequently, to be able to distinguish what brings joy from what brings suffering. The "school," which our karma has created for us in this world, teaches us the difference. That is, this "school," the world, which includes everything we can see, hear, smell, touch, or taste, or think about, truly exists for the purification of our soul.

"That which is to be eliminated is future sorrow," the great Yogi, Patanjali tells us in Yoga-sutra II.16. In other words, we do not have to suffer to be happy! While it is obvious when put this way, the presence of our karmic conditioning, in interaction with the five causes of suffering cited above, keep us in a state of amnesia regarding this truism. So, awareness is the ultimate reminder or "antidote" for our human forgetfulness. Only when we remember in every moment to stand as a Witness to our every action, word and thought, can we go beyond the "sorrow yet to come," resulting from our reservoir of karmas. We can stand back from the truckload of rotten tomatoes at our doorstep and say "Wow, look at that," and avoid getting so absorbed in "our problems" that we forget "I am not the problem," and "this too shall pass."

Is Divine Grace accessible to all? Yes, but only those who have prepared themselves know of its availability and aspire for it. "The Grace is equally for all. But each one receives it according to his sincerity," said to a great woman saint of the 20th century, and known simply as "The Mother." This requires that one cultivate non-attachment and equanimity in the face of the dualities of life: liking and disliking, having and not

having, getting and losing, pleasure and pain. Knowing that all is temporary, the wise remain always aware of that which is eternal and infinite, in
the midst of all changes. Whether their karma brings pain or pleasure, the
wise look upon them equally; they do not become excited or saddened by
either. As Jesus, said in the Sermon on the Mount, they lay not up their
treasure in places where mice can devour them, but in heaven. "For the
Kingdom of Heaven is within you."

So, the Divine Grace descends according to the degree of aspiration
and blossoming of the souls.

Question number 7: Can Awareness neutralize karma?

Awareness occurs whenever part of our consciousness separates itself
from that which is involved in the five senses, thinking or other movements of the mind, and standing back, merely watches. Awareness occurs
whenever we are fully present with whatever is occurring, and when we
choose to be the Seer, or Witness to the drama of our lives. One practices
various techniques or "kriyas" in order to cultivate such awareness in all
five planes of existence: physically through the physical postures of Yoga,
vitally through special breathing techniques, mentally, through various
meditation techniques, intellectually through the use of mantras, which
are sacred sound vehicles of consciousness and spiritually, through activities that cultivate love and devotion. It is the practical side of all religions.
A person's religion is a system of beliefs with regards to his or her relationship to a Supreme Being. Yoga is what that person chooses to do to
realize the goals of their religion. Most religious services, for example
involve the practice of what is referred to as *bhakti* yoga, the cultivation
of love and devotion for the Lord.

Awareness can lessen the effects of karma, because one can act in the
light of wisdom. One can reflect beforehand, and allow oneself to be
guided by a higher Self. Being fully present, centered and calm, one is
not swept away by attachments or aversions. On the other hand, in the
ordinary physical consciousness, one reacts to the forces of nature, acting
through various karmas, driven by habitual impulses. One continues to
create new karma as a result of attachments and desires and aversions.
Aside from karma, we are moved by three universal modes of natural
force, known as the *gunas*: action, inertia and balance. Because of our
ego, we all tend to personalize them, when we say, for example, "I am
tired" or when we feel the need to get up and do something. But we are

prompted and moved by these forces constantly. By practicing awareness, however one cultivates being "actively calm, and calmly active," reinforcing the presence in one's life of balance, equanimity, awareness, detachment, beingness, acceptance and love. This is an antidote to our karma, which acts through the other two major forces of Nature: activity, through attachment, with the feeling "I am the doer" and inertia, doubt, fear with the feeling: "I can't," "It's too hard," "I am afraid." By practicing the various "kriyas" of Yoga, one develops more and more the balanced mode of Nature within, and one becomes a master of one's life. One ceases to perpetuate karma; one exhausts old karmic tendencies. One realizes that one is an instrument, and that one is indeed, the Seer.

The above requires a systematic purification of the ego tendencies, and so awareness also involves self-purification of the over identification with the body, mind, personality, and a detachment from the ego's negative and contracting impulses. As a result, one realizes unconditional joy, or bliss, which is independent of whether one is getting or not getting what one desires, physically or emotionally. By slowing down, and being present in any given circumstance, one automatically becomes aware, and as a result bliss spontaneously arises. Being-consciousness-bliss becomes both the vehicle and destination because the Lord is characterized as Absolute Being, Absolute Consciousness and Absolute Bliss. Doing so, one realizes that the world is His self-manifestness. One realizes the Lord, and one transcends the Law of Karma.

The systematic practice of awareness thus becomes the master key to freeing oneself from the law of karma, and to realizing the ultimate goals of Dharma or righteous conduct: Self-realization and God Realization.

3. Liking and Disliking: the Disease of the Mind

As we deepen our practice of Yoga, we begin to realize just how much our mind is tossed about by things that we like and things that we do not like. We get excited, laugh or feel very "happy," when we obtain something we desire, or experience something pleasurable. We get depressed, frustrated, or anxious when denied what we desire. We encounter this throughout our day, at work, with our families, in the public, and in private moments. While we may long for the peace of our meditation cushion or asana mat, there is much that we can do elsewhere to overcome this "disease" of the mind.

Patanjali tells us in Sutra II.7 that "Attachment is the clinging to pleasure."

Because of the individuation of consciousness, and its false identification with a particular body and set of thoughts and memories, we are attracted to various pleasant experiences in our environment. Attachment *(ragah)*, like fear, springs from the imagination *(vikalpa)*. It occurs when we confuse the internal experience of bliss *(ananda)* with a set of outer circumstances, or factors, and we call this association pleasure *(sukham)*. We imagine that pleasure depends upon the presence of these external circumstances, or factors. When they are no longer there, we experience attachment, the delusion that the inner joy cannot return unless we again possess the external factors. Attachment involves clinging *(anusayã)*, and of course, suffering *(dukha)*. Even when we possess the external factors, we may still experience attachment because of the fear (imagination) of losing it. However, in reality, bliss is self-existent, unconditional and independent of external circumstances or factors. One need only be aware to experience it.

Patanjali goes onto tell us in verse II.8 that "Aversion (disliking) is clinging to suffering."

In the same way, we are repulsed by various experiences in our environment. These are relative terms, and what is painful for one, may be pleasant for another person. There is a third possible response however, detachment *(vairagya)*, which Patanjali proposes as the key practice for going beyond the painful and pleasurable (see verse I.12, 15).

When we go deep within, standing back from a painful experience, its cause becomes evident. By cultivating this perspective and understanding, as well as patience and tolerance, we are no longer troubled. "If it costs our peace of mind, it costs too much." Changing an outer painful situation is often impossible, without first changing our perception of it. We should first focus our will on clearing and deepening our consciousness to avoid reacting with aversion. Aspire for an outer change, for a more harmonious situation. Accept any work that has been given to you in the spirit of *karma yoga* (selfless service), as spiritual training, to purify yourself of attachment *(raga)* and aversion *(dvesa)*.

Both "attachment" and "aversion" are among the five afflictions, which Patanjali identifies in Sutra II.3: "Ignorance, egoism, attachment, aversion, and clinging to life are the five afflictions." These prevent Self-realization. Through ignorance of who we really are, we confuse the Self with the non-Self, the permanent, with the impermanent. Because of this ignorance, egoism develops. Patanjali tells us in II.6 that "Egoism is the identification of the powers of the Seer (*purusha*) with that of the instrument of seeing (*prakriti*)." In other words, egoism is the habit of identifying with what we are not, the body-mind personality, the instrument of cognition, as well as thoughts, sensations and emotions. We fail to recognize that they are objects, merely reflections of our awareness. This leads to the individuation of consciousness: "I-am-ness," and its confusion with "I am the body," "I am this feeling," etc.

This subject-object confusion can be removed by the practice of detachment and discernment. Feel that you are not "the doer," but only the "Seer." Be a witness and an instrument and notice how everything gets done.

To overcome "likings" and attachment, cultivate awareness before, during, and after pleasurable activities or circumstances. Notice that bliss remains throughout, as long as awareness is present. Practice letting go of the feelings of attachment. When things go well, thank the Lord.

To overcome aversion or disliking, perform all actions selflessly, skillfully and patiently. Cultivate equanimity as you perform all actions, and with regard to the results. When things go badly, take responsibility and learn to do better.

4. Doubts

One of the common tendencies of the intellectual part of our being is to allow itself to be invaded by doubts from time to time. Often they come at the beginning of ones career in yoga, or whenever there are challenges or failures in ones path. It is important to clarify the role of doubts, so as to use them constructively, rather to become their ping pong ball.

Patanjali tells us in Yoga-sutra I.31 that "doubt" is one of the nine obstacles to inner awareness. He says: "Doubt or *samsaya* is the tendency of the mind to question, and when it is not accompanied by a seeking of answers, it may leave one cynical and unprepared to continue to make efforts."

When the doubts motivate one to formulate clear questions, and then to seek answers, through meditation, or asking another person, they perform a useful role. In the beginning one is ignorant of many things, such as how to deal with different reactions of the body or mind, or vital, or ones increased sensitivity. Sharing with others helps one to find answers. It is useful to use the fourth or seventh meditation techniques, taught in Babaji's Kriya Yoga first initiation, particularly when one needs to go beyond emotional reactions associated with a doubt. So doubts can be good, if one makes an effort to seek answers. This begins by putting the doubt into the form of a clear question, and then seeking answers constructively. It may require that one do some reading. It may require that one exercise patience, waiting for the opportunity to speak to someone who may have the answer.

Too often, beginning students allow doubts to become "bad" by not communicating them constructively. They may simply become critical of what they have learned, or of themselves. They may complain or make judgments. They do not try to even form their doubts into questions and then to seek answers. Consequently, "bad" doubting causes them to stop their practice, out of confusion or discouragement. Even when it is very small doubt about how to do a particular technique, the student may not practice it, out of fear or confusion.

Too often people become cynical, and consequently they doubt just for the sake of doubting. A part of the mind can even take a perverse pleasure in indulging in the associated emotional feelings of doubt, such as fear, depression or anger. Much of our media is cynical, and it is easy to be infected by such cynicism.

One must also recognize the limits of understanding as we commonly know it. As Sri Aurobindo put it: "As for understanding, it is your physical mind (that part which works through the five senses and their subtle counterparts) that wants to understand, but the physical mind is incapable of understanding these things by itself - for it has no knowledge of them and no means of knowledge. All the physical mind can do is to be quiet and allow the light to come into it, accepting it, not interposing its own ideas - then it will progressively get knowledge... it must surrender...The mind in its higher part is aware of being one with the Divine in all ways, in all things - having the supreme knowledge, it is not disturbed by its own ignorance and impotence in its lower instrumental parts, it looks on all with a smile and remains happy and luminous." (Letters on Yoga, pages 1263, 1267).

So, doubts occur in the intellectual dimension of our being, often supported by emotions such as anger or discouragement in the vital. But by recognizing the game of the lower nature the wise soul remains undisturbed by them, and knows that truth itself cannot be expressed. One can only be it.

5. Sincerity

"In Babaji's Kriya Yoga, the only currency of any value is that of sincerity." This phrase, often repeated by my teacher, Yogi S.A.A. Ramaiah, provides a wonderful guideline for you in making your choices in life. The spiritual path is often littered with good intentions, which have been forgotten in the battle of life. To be sincere is to make your actions, words and thoughts agree. To be sincere is to follow through on your intentions, and to do what you say you are going to do. It is to determine what your priorities are, based upon your deepest values, and then keep them in mind when situations make demands upon your time and resources.

Sincerity has several components: a search for truth, a formulation of intention, a commitment to your intention, and perseverance.

1. The search for truth leads one to question and to reflect upon the meaning of life: Who am I? Why was I born? Where did I come from? What happens to me after I die? Is there a God or Supreme Being? If so, how can I know Him or It? Why is there suffering in the world? How can I overcome suffering?

The search for answers to such questions will lead you to read and study the great wisdom literature and sacred religious texts. But reading is only a beginning, and it will not change your human tendencies. It may point you to the next stage however, spiritual disciplines.

2. The formulation of intention is an expression of your will to find, to realize, to know. It is born from a recognition that you are no longer willing to go on without knowing the truth of things, without knowing unconditional love. It may also be born of a recognition that you are in a kind of prison as long as you do not transcend the ego's identities. It is born of an aspiration, a call of the soul to become one with That! As a result you make a commitment to a path, a religion, a spiritual discipline, or to God Himself. It is a promise, which must come from your heart. It may

be expressed in a formal ceremony, or in a personal moment of reflection and decision.

3. Perseverance, the third element required of sincerity is the sustained application of your will in the face of difficulties and suffering, to continue towards the realization of your intention. It is essentially endurance. You cannot give up. You must take the view that this is for life, and that apparent failures and stepping stones will lead to an eventual success. Human nature will resist due to its habits and its subconscious programming. Perseverance will continue to bring awareness and will, to bear, to "aspire, to reject resistance and ultimately to surrender to the process."

The practice of sincerity in the context of Kriya Yoga:

As a sincere practitioner of Kriya Yoga you will plunge daily into the depths of your soul and bring back the experience of the deepest values of Love, Peace and Truth. The intellect and mind will then translate these experiences into clear thinking and perception as we go about your tasks. To bring the body with all of its propensities and needs into alignment with your soul, the asanas must be practiced every day, with calm, soulful awareness.

To bring the emotions and the movement of various bodily energy currents into the service of the soul and psyche, practice Kriya Kundalini Pranayama and the allied pranayama techniques, remembering their Divine source.

To erode the ego's false identifications and attachments, its preferences, practice the mantras whenever possible, in the midst of daily challenges.

Then your life's thoughts, words and deeds will begin to flow as one current from your soul, connected to the Divine. They will express your sincerity and bring happiness to yourself and others.

6. The Eternal Smile

Life can often overwhelm us with concerns and distractions. It is not easy to see beyond the surface waves of change to That Eternal One. The example of enlightened ones can be illustrative.

My teacher Yogi S.A.A. Ramaiah was fond of recounting the story of "Chela Swami," a liberated soul and guru of his mother Thaivani Achi.

As a boy, his family estate was often visited by this holy sadhu who often behaved as a madman, wore no clothes, but who always had a smile on his face. Yogiar's mother would sometimes sigh and say, "it's so long since I've seen Chela Swami, I wander when he will come again." Within the next day or two, he would suddenly appear. Whenever he came, the neighbourhood children would turn their attention to him, considering him to be a simple "madcap." They would give him a banana, and he would smile, then someone would snatch the banana away from him, and he would smile. One of them would massage his feet, and he would smile. Then one of the naughty boys would kick dust onto him, and he would smile.

My teacher would end this story by asking his listeners "Why do you think he was always smiling?"

PART 2

Finding the Spiritual Path

1. Guru Purnima and the Guru

Tamaso ma jyotir gamaya

From the unreal lead us to the Real

From darkness lead us to the Light

From death lead us to Immortality

Gurupurnima is the festival where devotees celebrate the Guru. This year we celebrated it on July, 2004, at the Quebec Ashram. It was a magical night, with a full moon, pale yellow in color, on a balmy night. Later that night a terrific lightning storm came up and held us in awe.

Purnima means "full moon day." Guru Purnima is the day when the moon is the fullest of the whole year. It follows shortly after the longest day of the year, the summer solstice, usually in July.

"Gu" means darkness and "ru" means light. So Guru means "dispeller of darkness." Gurupurnima is the day when it is said that the rays of the sun touched the earth for the first time. It is the day of wisdom, the day of light.

Gurupurnima is the beginning of the spiritual year. It marks the beginning of *chaturmas*- a four month holy period of moderation and spiritual activity. On this day the aspirants offer their devotion and the fruits of their practice to the master in the form of their gratitude and love. Every disciple makes a new *sankalpa*, which is a pledge expressing their intention to practice more, to understand more fully the Guru's teachings, to do Guru Seva and to become worthy of receiving the Guru's grace. On Gurupurnima we seek the blessings of our Guru. Through concentration on the Guru on this day, through our mind, our prana, our Self, we can have a profound experience, or *darshan* of the Guru.

Who is the Guru?

The Guru is a spiritual preceptor, who initiates his disciples onto the spiritual path and guides them towards liberation. The Guru is one who has realized his identity with That, the absolute source of everything, and assumes the responsibility of guiding others to that realization. As such the Lord is manifested in the form of the Guru. For one who does not have a physical Guru, the Lord himself is the Guru.

A physical guru may merge with the Absolute Being Consciousness and Bliss, leaving the physical plane, yet will remain available and willing to help true aspirants. The Guru in subtle form remains however as the grace bestowing power of God. Guru, God, Self, all pervading consciousness, Shakti, all one. It is said, when a true disciple chants the guru mantra and meditates on his Guru, even if the Guru is not in a physical body, the Guru can feel the current of sublime thoughts coming to him from his disciple. The Guru responds to the vibrations of sublime thoughts in the wide expanse of superconsciousness and visualizes clearly a fine line of dazzling light between them. This is grace power light.

The Guru tattva or Guru principle is the principle by which Nature, creates, sustains and destroys all life in both our inner and outer universes, in whatever way is necessary for us pass from ignorance to wisdom, from egoism to Self-realization. Having existed before the universe was created it transcends time and space. The Guru principle exists within everyone as the inner Self, so when we honor the outer Guru, we also honor our own Self. It is the impersonal Shakti, the spontaneous force that creates whatever is needed for the greatest expansion of sadhana. It is more powerful than the external guru because it always accessible.

The Guru and the Gunas. The word "guru" is derived from the word "gunas." The gunas are the modes by which Nature manifests. They are three in number: *rajas,* or activity, *tamas* or inertia, and *sattva* or balance. The Guru is one who shows the aspirant how to overcome the influence of *rajas* and *tamas* and to become established in *sattva,* which is the entry for Self-realization. Ordinarily our human nature moves us back and forth between activity and inertia. We go through a daily cycle. Some of us may wake up in the morning filled with so much tamas (inertia) that we find it difficult to get out of bed. But after a shower, or drink water, coffee or tea, or do some exercise we begin to feel the force of activity. Nature moves us with universal force. When the force of rajas reaches its peak, we may feel great restlessness. Gradually, however, as the day progresses we begin to feel tired. By the end of the day when we are ready to go home, *tamas* or inertia predominates. Finally at the end of the evening we return to the state of sleep in which tamas predominates. Rarely are we in the state of *sattva*, or balance, which is characterized by feelings of calm, contentment, mental clarity, joy, love, and detachment. The Guru teaches us that Yoga has the effect of reducing the influence of *rajas* and *tamas*, and increasing the influence of *sattva* in our lives. The practice of our yoga postures and pranayama can energize and help us shake off feelings of inertia in the early morning. And yet, if done in the evening can help us to manage the effects of stress, such as agitation and nervousness and bring about restful sleep. They bring about balance and equipoise by ridding the body and mind both of excess inertia and restlessness. The practice of meditation and of mantras has similar effects on the vital and mental bodies. All of these practices promote homeostasis and equanimity, the pre-requisites for going within and becoming established in the perspective of the Self or soul, in the spiritual dimension. The Guru therefore can be experienced purely as "the teachings and wisdom" that comes through an acharya (teacher) of a lineage of Yogic techniques that leads us to the doorway of Self-realization.

Do You need a Guru?

With few exceptions, all souls which take incarnation in this world do so because they remain attached to duality. Notions of liking and disliking, getting and losing, high and low, good and bad, disturb us continuously. The identification with the body-mind is so strong, that they are drawn into the ego's snare of ignorance as to their true identity. Therefore, virtually everyone needs the grace and guidance of a guru, whether it is external or subtle, until and unless they realize the Self.

The Guru and the Guru's Teaching are one and the same. Real spiritual progress can only be made through applying the teachings. While reading spiritual books may point the way, they do not provide the essential experience or divine grace, which comes when one surrenders the limited ego perspective. Through practice of the sadhana prescribed by the guru, whether Karma yoga, the path of selfless service to the Lord, Bhakti Yoga, the path of devotion to the Lord, or Jnana Yoga or Raja Yoga, the paths leading to Knowledge of the Lord, progress must be made in overcoming the *samskaras* or habitual tendencies which bind one to the world of duality.

How do you know when you have found your Guru?

You should approach the Guru with profound humility, sincerity and reverence. You should have an eager and receptive attitude to the teachings of the Guru. If you find peace in the presence of your Guru, whether in physical or subtle form and find that your doubts disappear, then you should accept Him as your Guru. You should know, if you "accept" someone as your Guru that means He, long before, accepted you as a disciple. You would never have been able to accept Him without Him first accepting you. And know that you have found your Guru, if you receive answers, before you even verbalize the questions. You hear exactly what you need to know, when you need to know it.

Until that time, the best and perhaps only way of finding your Guru is by diligently preparing yourself. It is said, that when the disciple is ready, the Guru will appear, that is when your heart chakra opens. So apply yourself as a disciple to the yogic discipline and teachings of a Guru. See how you are affected. The Guru and the Guru's teachings are the same. A true Guru will emphasize the teachings, rather than his person.

Spiritual knowledge is handed down from Guru to disciples. The teachings of the Guru are called *Upadesh,* which means "near the place." The object of *Updesh* is to show a distant object quite near. The Guru makes the disciple realize that the Divine, Absolute Being, Consciousness and Bliss, which the disciple believes to be distant and different from himself is near and not different from himself. A disciple learns Yoga through dedicated practice of the teachings laid down by the Guru, by sincere self investigation and by service to the Guru.

The Inner Guru

While ultimately the disciple must one day transcend the external guru, and discover the guru as a spiritual principle or tattva within, in their hurry for enlightenment, Western disciples often discard the external guru prematurely, leading them to the risk of further confusion in the swamp of egoism.

The only inner guru accessible to the average individual is the ego-self. The ego-self is the cause of our un-enlightenment, and it pushes the disciple deeper into ignorance, confusion, self-delusion, and ultimately despair.

Powers of the Guru: the Guru may be understood by his powers and functions:

1. Guru as Initiator

The guru assumes responsibility for assisting the disciple's birth into the spiritual dimension, through the communication of esoteric knowledge, which initiates the liberation and illumination of the disciple.

2. Guru as transmitter

A Guru is a teacher who not merely instructs or communicates information, as does an *acharya*, but rather transmits wisdom, and by his very nature, reveals the spiritual reality. He initiates and even invigorates the spiritual process of the disciple. When the guru is not yet fully liberated, transmission is largely, but not exclusively based on the teacher's will and effort. Divine grace may also use such a guru as a vehicle.

Satguru is a fully enlightened guru, whose every word, gesture and mere presence is held to express and manifest the Spirit; transmission is extra-ordinary, spontaneous and continuous.

3. The Guru as guide

The Guru may guide through verbal instruction, as a living example, by oral explanation or commentary on the sacred texts, to yield their deeper meaning. The guru, by virtue of the oral transmission received from his or her own teacher or teachers, and also in light of his or her own experience and realization, is able to make written teachings come alive.

4. The Guru as illuminator

The Guru is the remover of spiritual darkness; restores sight to those who are blind to their own true Self. This depends upon the degree of the guru's own Self-realization.

5. The Guru as a disturber of convention

The guru swims against the stream of conventional values and pursuits. Their message is radical: asking us to live consciously, inspect our motives, transcend egoic passions, overcome intellectual blindness, live peacefully with others, and realize the deepest core of human nature, the Spirit. This disturbs those who are devoting their energies fully to the pursuit of conventional values.

6. Discipleship and the Guru

To benefit from the guru's transmission of liberating wisdom, one must enter into an intense transformative relationship with the guru that is known as discipleship. This includes a deep commitment to self-transformation, submission to a course of discipline, by which the mind is moved out of its conventional habit patterns, and a loving regard from the guru who must be viewed not as an individual, but essentially as a cosmic function. The guru is not interested in an interpersonal relationship, but to obliterate the illusion of discipleship, to draw the disciple into the realization of the supreme Self.

7. Authority of the Guru

This task of the Guru is effective with *prajna* (insight) and *karuna* (compassion) which are themselves supra-individual capacities oriented towards the Self, rather than the finite human personality. If the Guru is only compassionate, he could not guide the disciple out of illusion, and the disciple would misinterpret the compassion as love for how the disciple is now. The Guru loves the disciple in his true nature, the higher Self. If the Guru was merely wise, but lacking in compassion, most likely the disciple would become crushed under the demand for self-transformation. Disciples are prone to misconceptions, projections, illusions, and delusions that prevent or delay a constructive relationship with the guru.

Connecting with the Guru, Surrender and Grace

Yoga traditions describe various seats of the guru in the subtle system, the most powerful being the *sahasrara*. The guru is also inwardly heard in the forms of subtle sounds. The inner guru may be experienced without form, as Silence and the Infinite Spaciousness of the expansive heart. Our true inner guru lives in the *sahasrara* and is accessible and associated with our use of the mantra. The Siddhas favored form of initiation is to have the Guru's feet placed on top of the disciple's head. The Guru transmits his shakti through His mantra. The shakti enters the disciple when he chants his gurus's mantra. The mantra is a form of the guru himself.

Surrender is of critical importance. Surrender to the Guru will bring initiation, one way or another. Only through surrender can one unite with the Cosmic Being, and draw in immense grace. Grace removes all obstacles without which perfect union is not achieved. Surrender and grace are complementary to each other. The Guru has an infinite pool of spiritual energy received from the Supreme Being, which he can redirect to his disciples. Only the surrendered disciple can assimilate the powerful currents of spiritual energy that flows from the Guru, in direct proportion to the degree of his faith and devotion to the Guru.

Give Salutations to your Guru and to the Guru in all forms

Regard the Guru with deep love. It is important to keep the Guru in the heart, to be with Him/Her in principle and to keep attuned with Him.

- Salutations to the Guru, who is all pervading Pranava, the sound of "Aum."
- Salutations to the Guru, who is indicated by the term *sat chit ananda,* which means absolute being, consciousness and bliss.
- Salutations to the Guru, who is destroyer of all ignorance.
- Salutations to the Guru, who is established in supreme "I-consciousness."
- Salutations to the Guru, whose is the Grace-bestowing power of God.
- Salutations to the Guru, who is supreme knowledge, intellect, memory, delusion, cause and effect of everything.
- Salutations to the Guru, who made it possible to realize Her as the Universal Self, present in all beings and all beings existing in Her.
- Salutations to the Guru, who speaks to us with the small voice of our intuition.
- Salutations to our Guru, Kriya Babaji Nagaraj, who is the Guru of all Gurus, and who makes it possible for us to realize that our

soul is the soul of all beings.

- Salutations to Kriya Babaji again and again, who through His infinite grace and power, kindly leads His devotees from stage to stage and illuminates their latent physical and intellectual energies; who allows them to realize the transcendental physical enjoyment and supreme mental happiness, and ultimately leads us to His union with the Supreme Being. May His grace be upon us all.

Meditations on the Guru

- Chant your mantra and meditate on the form of the Guru you choose, and worship the sacred feet of the Guru. The Guru's feet are manifestations of the guru's energy in the subtle body. The feet or the sandals contain the liberating power of mantra.
- Keep your Guru's appearance and attributes fully in mind, and by reflecting on the same and affectionately following His teachings and instructions.
- Meditate on the Guru with form (*saguna*). Such *gurubhava* (devotion) is an effective way of strengthening the guru-disciple relationship. Meditate on the Guru, imagining him to be in every part of you. Let your body become filled with Him. Remember that just as a cloth is composed of threads, with cloth present in every thread, so are you in the Guru, and he in you. With this kind of vision, see the Guru and yourself as One. Let there be no difference between Babaji and you. Keep repeating in your mind, Guru Om. Implant the Guru in each part of your body, with a Guru Om, so that Babaji is within you.

2. Aspiration

"Rise up, prostrate, surrender, embrace, wonder;
Appeal in all the ways to the Holy feet of the Lord.
That brings the benefits of this birth;
Hold Him with reverence; He responds in turn."

- Tirumandiram, verse 1499

We are individually and collectively engaged in a process of transformation that requires a rejection of our old human nature and surrender to the Divine Conscious-Energy within. Although religion and Yoga both speak of the need for austerity, surrender to God's Will and Grace, the path and goal of Yoga is altogether different from that of religion. Unlike religion, the Yogin seeks not to depart from this world and to find some heaven, nor does the Yogin put faith in scripture or religious institutions above his or her own experience. Unlike religions, Yoga provides practical methods to experience truth and to master one's own nature. Yoga does not condemn our human nature as sinful, nor encourage its renunciation, but rather provides the means to purify oneself of ignorance, egoism, attachment, and all that resists the descent of Divine grace, while living in the world. Transformation is only possible when one has the knowledge of how to do it in this world. Only by being armed with this knowledge, will true aspiration, rejection and surrender allow the Lord's grace to descend and transform consciousness.

What is required for the descent of grace for the religious man and the yogi? In both cases what is required is the individual will, motivation and aspiration to reject what must be rejected, and to embrace and surrender to the Divine. Religion does provide a road map for man to follow, but not a tool case. Yoga offers the road map and also an arsenal of tools to facilitate the process.

How does aspiration differ from desire? Aspiration must not be confused with desire, for desires are always manifestations of the ego. The ego seeks to be separate, special, superior, and it manifests desires to strengthen its special-ness. Desires are the manifestation of the insatiable thirst and appetite of the separative ego-consciousness. But because of its inherent limitation in power and capability it cannot fulfill its urge to infinite and absolute possession. Hence there is an unbridgeable gap between its insistent demands and actual attainments. This creates constant discontent. Ego forgets that unless it drops the sense of separation the experience of divine unity and universality is impossible. For ego wants to possess the world without knowing it can be effected only in the spiritual way. So ego mistakenly follows its own impossible way, which amounts to gathering from outside, from what it feels as not-self, more and more objects of enjoyment to satisfy its ever-increasing hunger.

A genuine aspiration is just the opposite of this. It is intensely aware of the insufficiencies and imperfections of the ego-bound existence; hence it tries to release the hold of the ego's desires. Each movement of aspiration is directed not *to* the ego-centre, *but away from it*. And by this sole sign, a sadhak can recognize whether his or her governing impulse of the moment is of the nature of a desire or of an aspiration. Thus, an aspiration originates from the soul as a yearning towards the divine love, light, the beautiful, the good, the pure and progress. There is striving, even intensity, but without impatience or frustration.

How do I begin to develop aspiration? In stages, which usually begins with an intense dissatisfaction with the habitual ways of human nature. You wake up one morning and suddenly realize that you are no longer willing to go on living unconsciously, ignorantly, in a state in which you do things without knowing why, feel things without knowing why, live with contradictory wills, live by habit, routine, reactions, understanding nothing. You are no longer satisfied with that. Yet, how you respond to this dissatisfaction may vary.

For most, the first response from the soul is a need to know, for others it is what should I do to find meaning in my life? This questioning may lead secondly to ardent seeking to escape the entanglements of the world, in order to find Truth, Love, Peace, Joy, Being. Because these are at the most, very vague ideals, what we must do is to create change in the human personality plagued with ignorance and imperfections. Third, after some time, if we continue with persistent insistence, Divine Grace responds with a temporary piercing of the veil of ignorance, and we experience the spiritual dimension of life. We might see the Light, feel Divine Love, or experiences Divine Bliss, the Presence, or Truth, depending upon our capacity and orientation. This experience will vary from person to person, but regardless, everything else previously experienced in ordinary life will pale in comparison. Fourth, this new opening may close, so we must be careful not to forget the experiences, or to doubt them, but rather keep them vibrant and constantly direct our aspiration for their reemergence. Fifth, the sadhak will find that gradually his or her attraction to the higher life is growing and attachment to the old lower life is fading. This may manifest not only inwardly in the mental and vital planes, but outwardly with regards to friends, work and pastimes. A new type of yearning and resolution fills the heart and mind, which may express itself like this: "O Lord, I want you and you alone." In a sixth stage, the aspiration is so intense, that neither words or prayers, vocal or mental, are required. The flame of spiritual fire burns and rises steadily within a background of profound silence. An intense seeking to belong to the Divine becomes a desire for Truth, for transformation, for perfection.

As aspiration grows, Divine grace responds and introduces a higher determinism, a dynamism that can transform everything in our human nature. But for this to occur one must remember the following.

1. Be persistent and consistent. To aspire for an hour or two, and then to "forget" for the rest of the day does not get you anywhere. Keep the object of aspiration constant in your consciousness throughout your day.

2. Avoid impatience. This only brings doubt, unworthiness or rebellion.

3. Spend some time each day as the Witness. See the Divine in everything.

4. Consistently reject anything in your nature that tries to distract you and replace aspiration with desire.

3. Receiving the Grace of our Satguru Kriya Babaji Nagaraj

My teacher, Yogi S.A.A. Ramaiah, often cited three requirements to receive the grace of Babaji. "The amount of Grace you receive depends upon how much *sadhana* you do, how much karma yoga or service you do and how much love and devotion you manifest," he would say. Not only in words, but also in the ways he required us to live our lives, as residents of his ashram and centers. What exactly did he mean by the terms "grace," "*sadhana*," "karma yoga" and "love and devotion?" How were these teachings applied in the lives of his dedicated students? For now, a brief description can help Babaji's students find success in this field and in all five planes of existence.

Grace

"Grace" is a term one finds in many spiritual traditions, and it refers to all that we receive which helps us to evolve and to come closer to the Divine, ultimately experiencing our Oneness. It often takes the form of fortuitous occurrences, which we recognize as blessings, but it may manifest as blessings in disguise, cloaked in suffering as a result of some loss. It may also be experienced as spiritual experiences, such as Divine Light, visions, ecstasies or the descent of a great peace. Because it comes spontaneously, we attribute it to some force or entity outside of ourselves, usually the Divine form to which we are most devoted or allied with. As we often go through long periods where there is seemingly little progress in our spiritual evolution, despite all of our efforts, we seek the grace of the Divine to help us to reach new levels of awareness or experience. Both grace and effort are necessary for progress. Without our efforts to surrender our ego, there is no room for the grace in our lives. In ego consciousness we take credit for all the good things that come to us, and blame God for all the bad things. But when we awaken from the sleep of ego consciousness we realize that it is just the reverse.

My teacher often used to say: "All that is good is due to the Grace of Babaji, all that is bad is the work of the ego." Following its own selfish impulses of desire, as well as those of fear and pride, the ego creates a chain of actions and painful reactions. When, however, we purify the subconscious and awaken the consciousness of the Presence of the Divine, we become a witness and a consciously guided participant in His unfolding creation. The little promptings of the inner voice in the stillness of our soul are listened to and followed. The blaring trumpets of the ego, desire, fear and pride, are increasingly ignored.

To cooperate with our Satguru in this holy transformation of ego consciousness to Divine consciousness through Divine grace, *sadhana*, service and devotion are essential. What exactly do these terms mean?

Sadhana

"Sadhana" means "discipline," and it refers to all efforts to consciously remember the presence of God or to experience our true Self. One who practices yoga for these purposes is known as a *"sadhak."* A "Kriya Yoga sadhak" is one who follows the path of "Babaji's Kriya Yoga," practicing its techniques and following the teachings of Babaji. These techniques are taught during initiations and retreats. So are the teachings, which are also found to some extent in the publications released to date. Collectively these are referred to as "Tamil Kriya Yoga Siddhantham." As most of Babaji's teachings have been given in an oral form only, it will require a number of years before we can bring these out in the form of books and journal articles. Babaji's teachings are really the cream or condensed form of "Tamil Yoga Siddhantham," the teachings of the 18 Tamil Yoga Siddhas. The most important writings of which include "Thirumandiram," now published, (with a new edition with commentary nearing completion), Boganathar's collected works, (now translated and published), and Agastyar's collected works (which have yet to be col-

lected in their entirety, and translated). Babaji's two gurus were Bogana-thar and Agastyar, and so a complete understanding of his teachings will require that these be published one day. Rather than write himself, Babaji has preferred to crystallize the teachings he received from these two great Siddhas, or perfected beings, into "kriyas" or "practical yogic tech-niques," and to encourage their dissemination through dedicated souls whom he could use as instruments. One such soul was my teacher, Yogi S.A.A. Ramaiah, whose every action in life was soaked in the nectar of devotion for Babaji. He used to say, however, that Babaji could raise up any number of souls to the level of saints, sages and siddhas, if they would but surrender to Him. Another such soul was V.T. Neelakantan, who along with Yogi Ramaiah, founded the Kriya Babaji Sangah in 1952.

A Kriya Yoga "sadhak" is one who is consciously trying to surrender their ego consciousness for a Divine consciousness, by the systematic practice of the techniques and teachings of Babaji and the 18 Siddhas. "Kriya Yoga sadhana" refers to the practice of all of the techniques and activities prescribed in Babaji's integrated five-fold path: (1) Kriya Hatha Yoga, including asanas, bandhas and mudras for purification of the physical, (2) Kriya Kundalini Pranayama and related breathing tech-niques for the circulation of pranic energy in the vital body to bring about its transformation; (3) Kriya Dhyana Yoga, the scientific art of mastering the mind with all of its meditation techniques; (4) Kriya Mantra Yoga, the use of potential sound syllables to invoke the various aspects of the di-vine, awaken the chakras etc; (5) Kriya Bhakti Yoga, the cultivation of love and devotion for God and His creation.

By systematically practicing these five phases, the suffering caused by the ego consciousness gradually disappears and is replaced by happiness in all five planes of existence. For example, just by practicing Kriya Hatha Yoga systematically, we develop more radiant physical health, deeper relaxation and peace of mind. This new sense of health and peace liberates us from preoccupation with our physical body and its tendencies towards illness, inertia and pain. We are "freed up" to tune into the more subtle parts of our being and gradually free our self from mental emo-tional preoccupations, which like knots, bind us to rounds of painful ac-tions and reactions.

By practicing the Kriya Kundalini pranayama and other prescribed breathing techniques, you will experience tremendous amounts of energy, which can serve as fuel to overcome tendencies towards laziness, forgetfulness, and depression, when directed properly using Kriya Dhyana meditation techniques. Working together pranayama and meditation will help you to become increasingly aware of the Presence of the divine. Kriya Kundalini Pranayama brings more and more pranic energy up to the higher centers of awareness in the vital body: coincident with the heart, where it manifests as more and more love for God and others; at the throat center, with greater powers of self expression in various media; at the forehead center, where intuition, creativity, clairvoyance manifest; and at the crown center, where cosmic consciousness is realized so you experience the Presence of the Divine everywhere.

The practice of Kriya Dhyana Yoga purifies the subconscious and helps to replace habitual thinking and acting out with the very conscious awareness that you are being guided in all activities. It begins during brief moments during sessions of mediation when you become aware of your thinking or feeling, as the witness, and progresses to remaining aware during daily activities and even during sleep periods. You learn to be attentive and to discriminate and reject those habitual thoughts that are not helpful to remaining at peace. It leads you ultimately to the experience of samadhi, first experienced in the breathless state of communion with God, "sarvikalpa" samadhi, and if repeated often enough, during everyday life, as the continuous experience of God in everything, known as "nirvikalpa" samadhi. However, the ego, or habit of identifying with your thoughts, including your name, relationships, personal history, and ambitions, remains until you have completely surrendered all of your consciousness down to the last subconscious fear or desire, and down to the cellular level of your physical being. That requires a tremendous amount of *sadhana*, and until the ego is completely eradicated from your being it will continue to create mischief in all five bodies. As long as the ego is still present at some level of your being, you cannot experience the goal of "Tamil Kriya Yoga Siddhantham," which is "complete surrender" to the Divine. The hallmark of this complete surrender is *"soruba Samadhi"* wherein the cells of the physical body become, so to speak, "enlightened," or consciously directed by the Supreme Self. Divine Grace descends into all five levels of your being. When the physical body becomes ill or dies, even in the case of the greatest saints, it is an indication that at least their physical vehicle has not shared in their surrender and enlightenment.

Physical immortality is beside the point. Once you are completely surrendered, you will follow the direction of the Divine. But the possibility of complete surrender, the goal of Kriya Yoga, depends upon a realization of the Divine not just spiritually, as in the case of saints, or not even just intellectually, mentally and vitally as in the case of sages and siddhas respectively. Only the greatest of the siddhas, the so called "Maha Siddhas," as exemplified by the 18 Siddhas, and those of "Theosophy" can be deemed to have completely surrendered themselves to the Divine.

As a Kriya Yoga Sadhak you must gradually increase the time devoted to these practices and learn to integrate the awareness cultivated during them, into your daily activities. Meditation is not a goal in itself, but a means to an end. It should manifest with an increasingly awareness in each and every moment of life. All of your experience thus becomes a field for your practice of "sadhana" or remembrance of Self-awareness.

Karma Yoga

The meaning of the term "karma yoga" could be summarized by quoting the leading authority, Lord Krishna, Himself, who said "Do your duty, but leave the fruit of your action to me." During the initiation ceremony, one offers the fruit, remembering that these words apply even to our practice of the Kriyas.

Generally, people are motivated to do things because of the expectation of or desire for some personal gain, whether it be financial, notoriety or pleasure. But as the wise have discovered, desires just feed upon themselves, creating ever new desires, and locking one into a vicious circle of ever new desires. The end result is always suffering, whether one gets what one wants or not. If one doesn't, one becomes frustrated and confused. If one gets it, one becomes afraid of losing it, or it eventually loses its appeal and becomes boring. The Law of Karma says, "as you sow, so shall you reap," or "do unto others, as you would have others do unto you" to use a biblical paraphrase. Or, "do good, and good will eventually be done to you in measure; do bad, and you will receive in kind in due course." One cannot refrain from action as long as one is breathing, so Krishna advises us to do action that is our duty, not that which is based upon personal desire.

To gradually release the conditioning of action for personal gain, Babaji has asked his disciples to begin by setting aside several hours per week for "karma yoga" or selfless service. That is, to perform some service without expecting anything in return. This allows one to channel ones energies into a wider sphere, beyond the limited ego's desires, and to become a conduit for universal forces of love, which seek to work through us.

My teacher put a lot of emphasis upon this and got his students to meet every week for this specific purpose. During those years when we had many centers around the world, this karma yoga often included their maintenance or development. It also included efforts to publicize Kriya Yoga activities, poor feedings (particularly in India) and anything that would help the spread of Kriya Yoga. The personal effects were remarkable. One forgot about ones imaginary problems and became inspired and powerful in thought, word and deed. We were able to tap into a seemingly inexhaustible supply of energy and to realize many beautiful projects. In later years, these creations faded away, but that is another story. What was important was not what happened to the organization or its developments, but the development of Self-realization as the ego became dissolved by karma yoga, and the ability to be an instrument in the hands of the Master.

In karma yoga you begin as someone trying to lend a hand, or to do something in a selfless way, without expecting a payback. That is in the warm-up phase, so to speak. There is still two or more of us: "me" and "them." When you become a karma yogi, however, there is no doer. Out of the infinitely complex interplay of events and forces, things happen, and "you" are not the cause of any of it. Who you are, or who you thought you were becomes forgotten, leaving pure Being. "All that is good is the work of the Divine, all that is bad is the work of the ego," becomes Self evident. Of course, that little fellow, the ego, does not go easily. He goes kicking and screaming.

To give the ego a big kick, my teacher used to often keep us up late at night during marathon karma yoga sessions. Among other things, we would be sometimes asked to go outside at 2 a.m. to pull weeds (quite appropriate I now realize as a metaphor of the inner work also going on), for example - and that was before we could finally share the evening meal prepared hours before. Why? So the part of us that was tired and resisting would be released. Many people did not stay around him very long. In fact, few could stand the intensity of this practice. The first meditation technique and mantras came in very handy when the blood sugar became low and the ego started to rebel.

My teacher used to refer to the karma yoga to be done as "Master's work." This was a familiar expression for what is referred to in the sacred literature of Hinduism and Buddhism, as "dharma," that is your duty or mission in life. Your dharma is revealed as you go along, and becomes evident when you learn how to listen to the guide within. So, it goes hand in hand with all of the "kriyas," leading to "Kriya," or "action with awareness."

Why would the reception of grace depend upon how much karma yoga you do? It's not like anyone is keeping score of debits and credits, to see if you earn enough points to get through the pearly gates! Rather, karma yoga is the practical application of higher consciousness in ordinary circumstances generally ruled by subconscious conditioning. It is bringing love from the realm of meditation or devotional activities into the nitty gritty of human needs and transforming them. It is not service per se, for service can be done with an attitude, such as "how great or benevolent I am for doing..." It is, in effect, getting your personal desires out of mind at least out of the way for a while. It leaves space for the Divine to manifest, and thus to know your infinite Self.

Yoga is sometimes defined as "skill in action," and this is another important element of karma yoga. When something is done well, it generally means that it was done by someone who was fully conscious as to what they were doing. Undistracted by the petty desires of the mind, intelligence is able to channel itself intensely through the person, with force and inspiration.

Metaphysically, karma yoga also teaches you to act without creating any new karma. You cannot escape the effects of your past actions, but you can act consciously in any particular set of circumstances, without desire for personal gain, which would sew the seed for further karmic reactions. For example, if someone verbally abuses you, you can chose to react without losing control in anger or in a desire to inflict pain, and so avoid strengthening habits of getting angry or hurting others.

Begin to act in the spirit of karma yoga. Dedicate your actions to the Lord. Say "Om Tat Sat," which means, "I dedicate to Thee" whenever "you" complete something, receive your paycheck, do something nice for others. Expand the scope of your actions by doing volunteer work a few hours per week, allowing love to move through you and to use your gifts in ever expanding circles. Work selflessly to make Kriya Yoga known to others, to help us all to become liberated from the chains of ego formed karma. And remember, you are not the "doer."

Love and devotion

The yoga of love and devotion has been aptly described by Siddhar Thirumoolar in his "Thirumandiram," verse 270:

> "The ignorant prate that Love and Siva are two,
>
> But none do know that Love alone is Siva
>
> when men but know that Love and Siva are the same,
>
> love as Siva, they ever remained."

and in verse 274:

> "Worship the Lord with heart melted in love;
>
> Seek the Lord, with love
>
> When we direct our love to God
>
> He too approaches us with love."

and in verse 280:

> "What we scorned and what we gained, He knows;
>
> the righteous Lord in Love rewards as merit befits;
>
> Who, with burning zeal, seek Him with heart of love
>
> To such, well-pleased, He His Grace awards."

and in verse 283:

> "Like the sweet love in sex-act experienced,
>
> so, in the Great Love, let yourself to Him succumb;
>
> thus in Love sublimed, all your senses stilled,
>
> Bounding in Bliss Supreme, That this becomes."

and in verse 288:

> "The Lord God knows them who, by night and day,
>
> Seat Him in heart's core, and in love exalted adore;
>
> To them wise with inner light, actionless in trance,
>
> He comes, and, in close proximity, stands before."

This reminds us of the fact that mystics in spiritual traditions around the world agree on the fact that love is both the means to Self-realization and the end result.

How to cultivate such love and devotion for God?

By seeking ways to feel love towards others, be they divine forms, human beings, animals or plants. When you can meditate on the glory and greatness of God as an impersonal being, as *"sat chit ananda,"* "Absolute Being, Absolute Consciousness, and Absolute Bliss," you will feel blissful, and begin to identify with that. When you contemplate on the personal forms of the Divine, such as Jesus or Buddha or Babaji or in the form of His gods or goddesses, you also begin to identify, through love, with their divine qualities and essential nature. This may manifest, for example when you participate in spiritual or religious ceremonies, devotional singing or chanting, or visiting of holy places, where you view the images of divine personalities. You will become like that on which you most often think or meditate. Draw inspiration from these during the trials and tribulations of life to find the strength to overcome obstacles and the joy to keep a smile on your face. Interact with awareness and kindness with everyone with whom you come in contact, knowing that the Lord can be met at your very own door.

4. Discipleship or Devoteeship?

When a person feels drawn to a particular teacher or path and begins to absorb the teachings, one could say that such a person has become a "devotee." Such a person associates with others who feel similarly drawn to that path, studies its teachings, attends lectures and participates in activities organized to inform and inspire its participants. Doubts and questions may arise and the devotee seeks answers. It is sometimes a tumultuous period due to conflicts with old ways of relating or understanding, or because loved ones do not feel similarly drawn to the new path. The teacher may also test the sincerity of the devotee.

As one applies the teachings to ones life, and seeks answers to doubts, one gains assurance of their worth, and decides that the path is "right" for oneself. Or, one feels that it is lacking in something, and one continues to search. Like a ripening fruit, with experience in the path, color and sweetness manifest in the devotee; maturity and confidence develop. During this period one may be exposed to other teachers and teachings, and compare and test them.

However, at a certain point, one is ready to make the commitment to become a disciple to one teacher or to the teaching alone. A disciple is one who has made a commitment to surrender his entire being, heart, mind, body and soul to his teacher. Such a commitment is unwavering and for life. In the North American cultural context, where people are used to getting what they seek in as short a time period as possible - say two weeks, - whether it be fast food, clothes, reservations, relationships or enlightenment, few individuals are prepared to go through the process required to make such a commitment. Except when a self styled guru or "Maharaj" offers them enlightenment in a few months, if only they become his disciples. Especially if such a self-styled guru flatters their egos by giving them spiritual disciple names and puts them on stage for all to admire. Who could resist? It is easy indeed to be charmed by such a display. Sadly, after the infatuation fades, and the foibles and empty promises of such enlightenment salesmen are exposed, seekers become disillusioned. Such ex-disciples often bitterly express their disappointment and criticize their teacher, even though they were insincere "disciples." Who in the Western culture would get married before a courtship? Who would become a disciple before first becoming a devotee? Only in North America, where commitment to a teacher or teaching is generally an empty promise.

One should test and question a teacher and his or her teachings and allow plenty of time to pass before becoming his or her disciple. The guru should test the sincerity of his devotees by giving them the opportunity to face their doubts and apply the teaching before taking them on as disciples. Sadly, there are few true gurus and fewer true disciples.

Slow down, be patient, surrender even the desire for enlightenment, otherwise you could become prey to unscrupulous salesmen. You are That. Do not give it away.

5. The Significance of Initiation

In Babaji's Kriya Yoga the significance of initiation is often over-looked. Initiation is a sacred act in which an individual is given their ini-tial experience of a means to realizing some truth. That means is a *kriya* or "practical yogic technique," and the truth is a portal to the eternal and infinite One. Because this truth is beyond name and form, it cannot be communicated through words or symbols. It can be experienced however, and for this one needs a teacher who can share his or her own living ex-perience of the truth. The technique becomes a vehicle by which the teacher shares with the practitioner the means to realize the truth in one-self.

During the initiation there is always a transmission of energy and con-sciousness by the initiator and the recipient, even if the recipient is not aware of it. The transmission may not be effective if the student is full of questions, doubts or distractions. So, the initiator attempts to prepare the recipient beforehand and to control the environment so that these poten-tial disturbances are minimized. The initiator takes into himself or herself, in effect, the consciousness of the recipient, and begins to expand it be-yond its habitual mental and vital boundaries. There is a kind of melting of ordinary mental and vital boundaries, between the initiator and the re-cipient, and this greatly facilitates movement of consciousness to a higher plane. By so doing, he opens the recipient up to the existence of his own soul, or higher Self, which until then, remains veiled in the case of most individuals. By so raising the consciousness of the recipient, the latter has their initial glimpses at least of their potential consciousness and power. This is what is meant by the raising of the kundalini of the disciple. It is most often not done in a dramatic way in an initial session, but rather gradually over a period, depending upon the diligence of the student in putting into practice what he or she has learned.

For the initiation to be effective two things are essential: the prepara-tion of the student or recipient, and the presence of an initiator who has realized his or her Self. While most spiritual seekers emphasize the latter, and seek a perfect guru, few concern themselves with their own prepara-tion. It is perhaps a fault of human nature, to seek someone who will "do it for us." That is, give us Self-realization or God-realization. While the guru or teacher may point you in the right direction, the seeker must him-self commit himself to following those directions. While the seeker may be intellectually committed to following these, all too often, human nature causes one to waver in distraction, doubt or desire. So, even if one finds the perfect teacher, if one has not cultivated the qualities like faith, perseverance, sincerity and patience, the initiation may become as futile as sowing seeds on a concrete sidewalk.

Traditionally, for this reason, initiation was restricted to only those who had prepared themselves, sometimes for years in advance. While the first initiations may be made available to a larger number of aspirants, only those who had cultivated the qualities of a disciple were given the higher initiations. As Jesus said, "many are called, but few are chosen," only a few meet the demanding requirements of discipleship.

A devotee is one who is seeking a path or a teacher, and this may be for a very long time, until one is ready to make a commitment to one teacher or discipline. One may hop from one teacher to another, listening, watching, and experimenting a little, like a comparison shopper. At the end of that stage, one becomes a disciple, and becomes committed to the practice of the teacher's prescribed spiritual discipline. As the spiritual discipline requires persistent effort for an extended time for its results to be proven, one needs to have faith in the efficacy of the practice, perseverance, the support of a teacher, and divine grace. If the teacher is authentic, he or she will always be ready to respond to the student's request or to find someone who can. Divine grace is always available if one knows how to open to it. So, what is problematic is the faith and perseverance of the student. The teacher or guru can instigate the process through initiation and provide inspiration and encouragement, but the student must make the effort, with confidence and persistency.

If you were to learn the *kriyas* or techniques without initiation would they be effective? Understanding what has been discussed above, the answer is no. This is why trying to learn techniques from books or from teachers who have not themselves experienced the truth of which they speak leaves, the student uninspired. There is an essential sacred transmission of consciousness and energy, which occurs between the initiator and the recipient that empowers the techniques. That is why initiatory traditions have managed to pass the direct experience of truth from one generation to the next so effectively. Their strength lies in the power and the consciousness of those who have done the practices intensely and so realized their truth. We honor our highest Self when we honor our initiation by putting into diligent and regular practice what we have learned and received in them.

6. What is Babaji's Kriya Yoga?

About Babaji and his mantra

Om Kriya Babaji Nama Aum. One cannot begin to speak of Babaji's Kriya Yoga without mention of Kriya Babaji and his mantra, which has the power to attune one's pulse to the pulse of Babaji. This mantra can connect the heart of one's being to the heartbeat of the Universe. It can tune one into the grace of the legendary Himalayan *Siddha*, Kriya Babaji Nagaraj. Through it, He reveals Himself to His Devotees. Through the techniques of Kriya Yoga he guides the student in their sadhana and indirectly in their life. It is said that the inner guru abiding in the *sahasrara* is accessible and associated with the disciple's use of the mantra. The mantra is shakti, a powerful energy. The Guru transmits his shakti through the mantra and the shakti enters the disciple through the mantra. The mantra is a form of the guru. For the guru is a principle of nature, a *tattva*. And as such, it is force that creates and sustains life and directs the whole of the outer and inner universe. The Guru *tattva* transcends the limitations of time and space, for time and space are products of this creative principle and vital power.

The Guru principle existed even before the universe was created, and just like the elements of water, earth, air, fire and ether, it has been apart of creation ever since. The Guru principle is within everyone as the inner Self. When we chant the mantra we are giving respect to this inner guru, paying respect to our very own Self. The Guru is the Self, which is supreme consciousness and supreme bliss.

Explanation of the Mantra OM KRIYA BABAJI NAMA AUM

Om is pranava, the sound which runs through the prana.

Kriya is one of the three kinds of shakti or energy: that of action o*r kriya* shakti; that of will or *iccha* shakti, and that of wisdom, or *jnana* shakti.

Babaji is the living fountainhead of Kriya Yoga, its Satguru, the form of the Lord as The Father ... the same Babaji who was described by Paramahamsa Yogananda in his "Autobiography of a Yogi."

Nama is "salutation" or "my name is"

Aum is the sound of the universe inside yourself. Nama Aum is a call or a prayer to That highest Self, the *Satguru*.

As you become more aware of the Self and the Supreme Self, the hand or at least a finger of the Lord is felt in all circumstances. You begin to get sight of the Lord. You begin to feel your self being directed, being accepted. As you establish a perpetual relation with the guru you become guided in whatever work the *Satguru* gives to you to do. This is "Kriya Yoga."

The Origin of this Kriya Yoga Tradition

Kriya Babaji is a great yoga master who has lived for centuries in Tibet and in the Indian Himalayas in relative obscurity from the outer world. With the publication of *Autobiography of a Yogi* in 1946, Paramahansa Yogananda brought Babaji's existence to the attention of a wide audience. According to Yogananda, Babaji has exercised, mostly anonymously, an enormous uplifting influence as He works through countless others.

In fact, Yogananda cites Babaji as the master who, in 1861, initiated Lahiri Mahasaya into the Kriya Yoga techniques that brought him to Self-realization. Lahiri in turn initiated Sri Yukteswar, who subsequently revealed the techniques to Paramahansa Yogananda, who then brought this knowledge to the West. In 1920, he founded the Self-Realization Fellowship, and since his passing in 1952, this organization has faithfully continued to disseminate his teaching through books and a correspondence course.

This tradition of Babaji's Kriya Yoga flows directly from the ancient Kriya tradition of India, from perfected masters of Siva Yoga, known as the Eighteen Siddhas. Babaji himself had two principle gurus, Agastyar and Boganathar. The book *Babaji and the 18 Siddha Kriya Tradition* provides the details which Babaji has chosen to reveal about early life with these great Siddhas. This book, as well as another, which was dictated by Babaji in 1952 and 1953, to a disciple known as V.T. Neelakantan, published today with the title *The Voice of Babaji: Triology on Kriya Yoga*, also reveals the early years of a new mission which Babaji started through his instruments: V.T. Neelakantan and S.A.A. Ramaiah.

Babaji's Kriya Yoga includes 144 Kriyas or techniques, which form a progressive system, traditionally taught in a series of initiations over many years. This particular five-limbed Yoga system was specifically taught to Yogi S.A.A. Ramaiah, directly and in person by Babaji over several months in 1955 near Badrinath, in the Himalayas. The first initiation includes the very important technique of Kriya Kundalini Pranayama, which is quite similar to the technique taught by the SRF today. Paramahamsa Yogananda, spoke of the practice of Kriya Kundalini Pranayama as a means to accelerate the natural progression of Divine Consciousness in human beings.

In 1983, Yogi Ramaiah, or Yogiar, as he was known, began to prepare one of his students, Marshall Govindan, to teach the 144 techniques with a stringent set of conditions to fulfill. M. Govindan had by 1983, already been practicing Kriya Yoga at least 56 hours per week without a break for more than twelve years, an ideal period of which Yogi Ramaiah had often spoken. In addition, in 1981 Govindan completed a year long silence in retreat, alone, in a hut by the seashore in Sri Lanka, engaging in a non-stop practice of Yoga. It took Govindan three more years to fulfill the additional conditions, at which time, Yogiar told him, "now, you wait." Yogiar often said that once he had brought his students to the feet of the "Guru," his work with them was done. On Christmas Eve, 1988, in a series of profound spiritual experiences, a surprising message was given by Babaji to Govindan to leave his teacher's ashram and organization and begin initiating others into Kriya Yoga.

Henceforward, Govindan's life was directed by the continuous and inspirational Light of the Guru, and it focused on showing the path to others. Beginning in 1989, his life moved in this new direction; doors opened automatically, and everything facilitated a new mission. In 1992 Govindan founded Babaji's Kriya Yoga Ashram in Quebec. In 1997 he founded the lay order of teachers or Acharyas, known as Babaji's Kriya Yoga Order of Acharyas. It is now a tax exempt, educational charity registered in Canada, the USA, India and Sri Lanka. To date, there are more than fifteen teaching acharyas in a dozen countries. The Order has also since 2000 sponsored the research, preservation, transcription, translation and publication of the writings of all of the 18 Siddhas who are at the origin of Babaji's Kriya Yoga, as well as *The Voice of Babaji: Trilogy on Kriya Yoga.* Babaji's Kriya Yoga is a vehicle that can enrich life and can take anyone toward the ultimate goals of life, Self-realization and God realization. These precious texts serve as a necessary roadmap for this vehicle.

What is the goal of Babaji's Kriya Yoga?

Kriya Yoga enriches life. It strengthens the body, mind and soul. Its various practices work to make the practitioner healthy and to strengthen the nervous system. All sense perceptions become keen and clear, the mind and intellect are wonderfully sharpened. Man's latent faculties are developed and personal power is increased. The kriya yogi however, does not develop more energy and personal power for his own personal interests, but instead to become a more useful member of his or her community. Kriya Yoga is not for renunciants but for those who wish to serve and help humanity itself.

Yoga is a practical science of living a spiritual life. Kriya is "action with awareness." Therefore, Kriya Yoga has to be attained in and through activity, not only in so-called yogic practices but in every day living.

Babaji speaks of his Kriya Yoga in the Voice of Babaji:

"Sadhana should not imply a divorce and severance from normal life. The latter will itself become a dynamic sadhana through a shifting of your angle of vision. A proper bhava becomes the philosopher's stone to transfer the normal into the yogic. The eminently practical nature of Kriya Yoga renders it the rational bridge between the idealism of pure philosophy and the hard realism of earthly life. Its claim upon modern man is that it strikes a golden mean between the entirely abstract speculations of the mere theorist, and the overdone matter-of-fact attitude and the prosaic hard-headedness of the rank materialist. It is concerned with the transcendental life, yet asks you to take nothing for granted. You are to follow definite methods, arrive at tangible results and experience them in your own life. Its scope is comprehensive. It aims at an integral development of all faculties in man. It is then the precursor and the direct herald of the race of supermen into which present man has to evolve. It has as its aim, the creation of a new man of deep illumination and high vision and the establishment a new world order, a satya yuga, world of truth, as a result of such enlightenment.

The modern world abounds in conceptions of Yoga ranging from the deeply mystic and sensible to the absurd and ludicrous. Conflicting views and wild fanciful notions have clustered around conceptions of Yoga and sadhana. It has become conventional to conjure a picture of an emaciated, half-naked, ash smeared figure with matted locks, seated cross-legged beneath a spreading tree. Through long associations as well as mischievous misrepresentations, such notions have taken deep root. The superphysical phenomena occurring in the practice of Yoga and practitioner's experiences on subtler planes are viewed with suspicion and regarded as magic. Now this point is to be grasped clearly. Kriya Yoga is neither fanciful nor does it contain anything abnormal. It is not for the favored few. It is not a strange unnatural process practiced by a small minority to gain some strange or extraordinary end. Kriya Yoga is a time-tested, rational way to a fuller and more blessed life, which will naturally be followed by one and all, in the world of tomorrow. It is not dependent upon the possession and exercise of any abnormal faculties. It only requires you to develop faculties that you already possess but which are lying dormant within you. The chief instrument that it utilizes is one that is common to the whole of humanity, namely, the human mind.

Kriya Yoga is thus, not a study or practice meant only for the reclusive in the Himalayan caves. It is not only meant for one who clothes himself in rags, who has the stone as the pillow, who eats what he gets by a mere stretch of his two palms, who weathers the cold and the heat, who remains under the canopy of the sky. Kriya Yoga is meant equally for those who live in their different stations in life, who live in the world and who live to serve the world. It is not only a property of the samnyasin, or the yogi, but is also a universal property. It is a universal subject that requires deep study and sincere practice at the hands of citizens, townsmen, villagers and forest-dwellers. It is the marvelous science whose one fruit is not of discord, but of true peace, born of the soul, born of Infinite Bliss."

"Kriya Yoga, in even the smallest detail has the unique advantage of innumerable multiplications, from age to age and man to man. The verbatim and literatim sameness of these methods is Kriya Yoga's greatest point."

"There is a certain sacredness and superbness and purity about methods that are 'untouched by human hand,' when it has to deal with millions. There remains no room for discussion or the smallest doubt about the purity of the methods. The highest importance of the Vedas and scriptures arises not only from the most invaluable truth and wisdom con-

tained therein, but from the guarantee that they carry a purity of being 'untouched by human hand.'"

Svadharma: our reason for living

The ultimate goal of all of us is the same thing. What "seekers" are most aspiring for in life is permanent happiness. Non-seekers are looking for that happiness by temporarily satisfying desires. Seekers see through that temporary happiness and are looking for something else, something more. They know that their dissatisfaction with the fulfillment of desire comes from their inner being, that their inner being is turning on the pressure and pushing them towards their *svadharma:* their duty, their responsibility "to know thy self," "to be true to the Self," "to know what they came to learn and to do."

We are born into this life and most of us take it for granted that we are here never delving very deeply into the meaning of our existence. Yoga says that there is one single reason that we are on this earth and that is our *svadharma.* And our *svadharma* is not really to be happy. The reason we are here is to know our self and to be true to our self. To know who we really are and to let go of what we are not. Therefore whatever we can do to acquire the knowledge of who we are and let go of what we are not, is important *sadhana.* That is what Babaji's Kriya Yoga is assisting us in doing. It is said that we are all progressing in that direction whether we are conscious of it or not. However with a daily *sadhana*, pranayama, meditation, Hatha yoga, with constant practice, self study and devotion to the Lord we will progress more rapidly.

According to Hinduism there are four goals of human purpose: first, to obtain wealth, second, to obtain pleasure in physical comfort, emotional well-being and intellectual stimulation, third, to live a moral life, and fourth, self-realization or liberation. Babaji's KriyaYoga can assist us in all these four goals. For Babaji's Kriya Yoga is a spiritual tradition designed to wake us up and lead us on this path of self-realization. But it is also a comprehensive practical discipline and an open-hearted approach to live life fully. This tradition flows directly from the siddhas, the perfected masters of Siva Yoga. The techniques were developed by *siddhas*, perfected masters who were often householders, not renunciants. They had spouses and were socially conscious wanting the well-fare of humanity and often supported humanity with scientific and medical discoveries.

The Siddhas who developed this scientific art of Kriya Yoga have a famous saying: "the amount of happiness in life is proportional to one's discipline." Discipline in the context of Kriya Yoga, is doing what is required to remember who we are and to let go of what we are not. It is based upon the *siddhas* diagnosis of our human condition. They say that "we are dreaming with our eyes open." The world appearance only seems to be existent. Life is a dream, it is transient, and everything comes and goes like dreams: All of years of: acquiring experiences, possessions, respect, humiliation, bad times, wonderful times, relationships... all come and go like dreams.

Furthermore, Kriya discipline begins with the cultivation of awareness. But, most of what we do normally is done unconsciously, out of habit, without awareness. When we are awake to the world we are not awake to who we are, which is Awareness itself. When we are awake to the world we are not aware of the movement of our thoughts through consciousness. But, we accept the pleasure and pain they bring.

When we are awake to the world we are not aware of the movement of prana (the bioplasm or vital life energy in the body), but the mind gets agitated and the senses get stirred up and the mind gets agitated only when and if the prana becomes blocked or resisted in the body. The agitation and resistance of the life forces is due to mental confusion and this confusion can cause disturbances in the metabolism in the body. Mental confusion can cause foods to turn into poisons. Physical disease can occur.

Continual awareness of the activity and actions of the body, mind, and emotions can remedy mental and physical disorders. This practice of awareness can calm the mind and regulate the *prana*. "Action with awareness" is the definition, the vehicle and the destination of Babaji's Kriya Yoga.

Okay, so what is Awareness and how do we attain it? Awareness occurs whenever part of our consciousness is standing apart and witnessing what the rest of our consciousness is involved in doing, feeling, or thinking. This rarely occurs in the ordinary course of life, because usually we allow our consciousness to be absorbed by objects of attention, such as what we are seeing, hearing, and thinking or doing or we allow our consciousness to be dispersed in many different directions. When was the last time you watched yourself watch a sunrise or watched yourself read a book or watched yourself become angry or watched yourself do a Hatha Yoga posture? Rarely do we go inward to watch ourselves do anything.

And what does this sense of awareness do for us? As we allow ourselves to rest inwardly more and more, we become detached, so that the mind becomes calm in all situations and the prana becomes calm and regulated in all situations and the mind becomes purified and happiness and contentment arises in the heart. This is the goal of Kriya Yoga in a nutshell.

Kriya Yoga is an integral Yoga: a five-fold path for integrating the five bodies

Kriya Yoga will work on all parts of your being, and it can literally change your outer nature. It can change what you are doing in life and what you thought you were even capable of doing. It develops your potential. It is dynamic and transformational Yoga.

An integral Yoga is one which comprises all parts of the being and all the activities of the being. But, what we find is that the practices for one person will not be as powerful or as integral as the same practices are for another person. This is because we are not all integrated to the same extent. To be integrated we have to prepare all levels of our being.

The body is a temple of divinity. It expresses the Spirit. It is not only for living a physical and mental life. But most of us are just living physical/mental lives, so we have to educate our body to develop our spiritual faculties. We must systematically develop our spiritual being as we remedy our physical, vital, mental, and emotional defects and shortcomings to acquire intellectual abilities and a more balanced emotional nature. This is possible only when all levels of our being participates in a regular daily Yoga practice.

Babaji's Kriya Yoga is a genuine system to bring about awareness and Self-realization. It is founded in a set of 144 techniques. It is a five-fold path of asana, a specific series of eighteen *asana*; specific *pranayam* techniques, specific techniques of breathing, which directs prana and consciousness in the body; specific *dhyana* or meditation techniques to develop strong mind and inner senses, strong visualization skills and a means of actualizing those visualizations; specific *mantras* to awaken the intellect to its potential energy and consciousness and *bhakti*, love and devotion to invoke the "grace of God." *Bhakti* is required to develop the steadfastness and firm ground necessary for one to control the senses in such a way as to control the ego desires and aversions that arise through them.

The Objectives of the Five fold path

Kriya Yoga is "Action with Awareness." It is a means of self-knowledge, of knowing the truth of our being. Babaji's Kriya Yoga incorporates awareness in the practice of asanas, pranayama, meditation, mantras, but, also teaches to incorporate awareness in all thoughts, words, dreams and desires, and in all actions. This sadhana has the enormous potential to make us more conscious human beings. It requires, however, the willingness of the body, mind, heart and will, to align with the soul in aspiration of purification and perfection. The sadhana of BKY is a collection of exercises and spiritual practices for self development, but, it is also a way of life for our entire being.

The first objective of **Kriya Hatha Yoga** is deep physical and mental relaxation. Asana deals directly with the material part of the physical totality. Through the 18 asana the body becomes purified of many disorders and irregularities. The physical nervous systems becomes strong and the mind calm. The variety of asana grants flexibility and a sense of lightness and buoyancy in the body, so that gravity has less an effect on it.

The regular practice of this series of postures will help you conquer the distractions of the body and deepen meditation. Practicing the eighteen postures will slowly liberate you from inertia, restlessness, pain and illness. You will feel less physical and mental fatigue and when tired, more easily recharged. You will begin to tune into the more subtle parts of your being and develop awareness of the movement of energies in your body and learn to direct those energies. Asana, bandhas and mudras build a strong foundation for meditation. You will be more stable and at ease sitting for meditation in comfort and ease. Ultimately, the practice of Kriya Hatha Yoga readies the body, mind and nervous system, strengthening the subtle nervous system, stimulating the subtle energy centers along the spine and uncoiling and stimulating the upward movement of *kundalini,* thus, awakening potential power and consciousness.

Kriya Kundalini Pranayama, the scientific art of mastering the breath and the mind is the most potential technique in Babaji's Kriya Yoga. It is an elaborate yet powerful breathing exercise to connect prana and mind. It has the power to gently awaken *kundalini* (our potential power and consciousness), and to circulate it through the seven principal chakras located in our vital body, from below the base of the spine to the crown of the head. It awakens the chakras' corresponding psychological states and increases dynamism on all five planes of existence.

Pranayama had the greatest importance in the Yogic training of the Siddhas. Pranayama is a means to longevity, but it is also a means of obtaining an inner vision of the Lord.

Irregular breathing negatively affects one's health and leads to early deterioration of the body's constituent elements. Regular practice of pranayama is imperative if decay of the physical body is to be overcome.

The first objective of pranayama is to purify the nervous system and to balance and circulate vital energy (prana) throughout all the nerves and energy channels (nadis) without obstruction. Ultimately, the pranayamas of Kriya Yoga will balance the flow of the breath through both nostrils and the subtle nadis. This is turn will balance and steadiness to the subtle pranas. Pranayama helps the mind become more peaceful and steady, which helps us attain dharana (one-pointed concentration) so that dhyana (meditation) can happen. Kriya Kundalini Pranayama opens the central energy channel, (sushumna) and gathers more vital pranic energy into it, directing it upward stimulating the higher centers of awareness in the vital body. The techniques of Babaji's Kriya Yoga are taking us far beyond our normal range of consciousness.

Babaji's Kriya Yoga Dhyana, the scientific art of mastering the mind, demands that the truth realized in our inner consciousness will penetrate to our waking consciousness and become effective there. Our consciousness determines the nature and quality of the life we live. So, rather than trying to stop thoughts and drop into a void, our meditations focus on dynamic methods to strengthen the power of the mind and stimulate a ready flow of intuition and inspiration applicable to our life's challenges and mission. These unique *dhyanas* or meditation techniques help us to develop our power of concentration and visualization for orienting the whole of our consciousness in all its parts toward the aspiration of our soul. Ultimately these meditations lead to awareness of our true Self.

In a progressive series, each meditation builds on each other and helps to develop another level of consciousness. They have the ability to reach and affect all five bodies and different levels of our consciousness: the subconscious and unconscious, mind, the intellect and even supra-consciousness. They take us through a process where we are encouraged to become consciously aware of our mental conditioning, our desires, aversions, and cravings and then to consciously abandon them. They work to develop our inner sensing and open us to the flow of intuition. The practice of Kriya Dhyana Yoga purifies the subconscious and helps to replace habitual thinking and acting out with the very conscious awareness that we are being guided by our higher Self in all activities. (This begins during brief moments during sessions of meditation when we becomes aware our thinking or feeling and then follows us in our daily routines and we develop awareness of being guided in our actions and reactions in daily activities and sometimes even during periods of sleep). Through these meditations we learn to be attentive and to discriminate and detach from the thoughts which are useless or negative, which obstruct our peace and happiness, and learn to replace them with constructive positive movements and actions.

Man is very creative. How often are we told, "as a man thinks, so he becomes." We can create out of nothing the things we imagine. We have great imagination and powerful projection. These dhyanas develop and utilize that great power of imagination. Imagination can travel ahead of life, for imagination is the capacity to project one self outside of realized things and toward things that are realizable, and then draw them to us, through projection.

Ordinarily we use our imagination badly, imagining the worst that could happen (fear) or imagining the worst about others (judgment) based on limited information, or by imagining how good something would be (desire) or how bad something is (aversion). Take worry for instance, we all do it. Isn't worry just meditating on what we don't want? Why not imagine the most positive things in life? Why imagine catastrophes, when we could just as well imagine positive and healthy outcomes in life?

Imagination is an instrument that must be disciplined. Imaginations which are built up realistically and consistently with detail and aspiration or desire have a tendency to come about. When we add vital life energy to the process it becomes a living force. Most of our imaginings aren't very steady and don't have vital life energy behind it, because we usually lose interest and move on onto another imagining. Well formed imagining with aspiration, faith and trust, after some times are realized. The Kriya Dhyanas provide the discipline required to direct and reorient imaginings toward the goal of life. Several of the meditations specifically develop our imagination in order to create a new reality.

Kriya MantraYoga keeps ones' whole being calm, and consciousness tuned toward the soul. The *bija* or seed mantras, which are taught in Babaji's Kriya Mantra Yoga open us to the divine forces of ascending energy (kundalini shakti) through the chakras, and the descending grace. There are also specific mantras that cultivate development of the divine qualities, love, compassion, kindness, insightfulness, discipline and endurance. Mantras take your attention off the sense of "I" and "mine," and on the Lord within and without.

Kriya Bhakti Yoga is the cultivation of aspiration for the Lord Himself, or formless Truth; union with the absolute and liberation from the prison of ego identification, desires and attachment. Ultimately it is "love of God" that must root out lust, anger, desires, pride and envy to gain heavenly bliss and joy in life. It is the sense-desires, not the Lord, which leads us on the path of pain and suffering. Bhakti is a means of understanding that we need to possess nothing, but instead be a witness to everything. Bhakti helps us to understand that we are merely beads strung on the thread that is the Lord Himself. That thread never breaks and we are never scattered. Bhakti is a means of both uniting with and serving the Lord within and without.

Kriya Yoga requires Self-study

To practice Babaji's Kriya Yoga sincerely, you must be willing to study your self. By exerting yourself repeatedly, you can make change in both mind and personality. Babaji's Kriya Yoga is a concentrated daily practice of purification, which can be undertaken to rid yourself of your weaknesses and shortcomings and can help you to reach a place of peace and inner prosperity.

A disciplined daily practice of Babaji's Kriya Yoga creates an internal heat, which helps to burn away the distinctions, the mind and body has established, relating to its likes and dislikes, its aversions and desires, its discomfort and pleasure. One can change any habit of responding in a negative way, or create a positive attribute, by doing the practices over and over again. Once the practices of Kriya Yoga are no longer an exertion, but simply a way of life, then also, a new positive perception and attitude will have become a new way of living it.

A Discourse on Prana and Pranayama

Pranayama is not deep breathing. Ordinary breathing through the nostrils is one phenomenon. The movement of prana through the subtle body is another, which is vastly more important. Pranayama is not about absorbing more oxygen into the body, it is about connecting prana with mind, it is about learning to restrain and direct both prana and consciousness in the body. Prana is vital life energy, the bioplasm of life. Prana is the dynamic counterpart to the coiled kundalini.

The siddhas studied the flow of air through the nostrils and correlated it with the flow of prana in the *ida, pingala* and *susumna nadis*. They discovered that the flow of prana in the body is also influenced by the cycles of the moon and sun and that prana flows through the nadis normally in a synchronized manner with the solar or lunar cycles, or to specific circadian rhythms in the body. When the moon changes bimonthly with an ascending and descending cycle, the nadis also change dominance. The left nostril dominates in ascending lunar cycle (bright half of month). The right nostril dominates in the descending lunar cycle (the dark half of the month). That is, during the bright half of month the left nostril dominates at sunrise on the first, second, seventh, eighth, ninth and fourteenth days, and full moon days, but in the same cycle the right nostril dominates at sunrise during the remaining days. But still nostril flow alternates nostril about every two hours.

The term pranayama is derived from two words, "prana," which means energy and "ayama," which is also a composite of two words meaning to "stretch like a bow." It means development and extension. "Pranayama" is therefore a process of gathering energy together and directing it to remove blockages in the vital body, the *pranamaya kosha*. This process helps us to gain mastery over inner pranic forces, which helps us gain mastery over the body and mind.

The Siddhas call pranayama an "inner agnihotra" (a sacrificial fire) and promote the practice of pranayama as "a daily sacrifice in respiration" to that fire. They see it as a source of purification of the mind, body and desire. Pranayama aims at control of the mind. Pranayama will immediately relax both body and mind as it increases the amounts of energy, which, when directed properly can serve as fuel to overcome tendencies toward laziness, forgetfulness and depression. Once the prana is fully controlled, mind is fully controlled and so thought processes and emotions can no more cause us disturbance because we are able to control our temperament, moods, desires and aversions. We become more and more aware of the natural fluctuations of the mind.

Pranayama develops the gross outer and subtle inner Prana. As the outgoing and ingoing breaths are harmonized we contact the inner Prana and experience a sense of lightness, ascension and expansion. Prana is what heals the body and mind. Pranayama purifies and energies the body for the higher meditation which follows. "Prana" is the vital force and "ayama" is expansion so pranayama is the expansion of the vital force. One slows down and extends the breath so that the inner Prana or higher life force can manifest. This aids in slowing down and calming the mind, facilitating meditation.

Every psychological state has a corresponding rate of breathing. The brain wave patterns change with the presence of the breath in the body. Shallow breathing creates beta brain waves, where as abdominal breathing creates alpha brain waves. It is due to the restlessness of the breath that the mind moves from one object to another. Alpha brain waves are rhythmic and indicate that the brain is in a calm and relaxed state of wakefulness. They activate healing energy and meditation and are involved when we are states of euphoria. The body and mind automatically reacts to the deepening breath. Controlling our breath through pranayama concentrates our mind. Concentration, clarity, memory and creativity are often enhanced by these pranayams.

Kriya Kundalini Pranayama techniques are a process of "awareness training." Pranayama always involves awareness; breathing exercises do not. We must be fully attentive to what we are doing internally, so that we can enter into awareness. Attention brings the conscious brain (neo-cortex) into action and keeps one in a state of awareness. Awareness begins with attention. When done twice daily, Kriya Kundalini Pranayama builds a wonderful foundation for continual growth in a yogic awareness. In combination with the meditations, they can bring the necessary balance and growth to our personalities; whether that means you develop more critical thinking, or more feeling in the heart or intuition. The key to success in pranayama is in being totally involved in the doing of them.

The Subtle Body: nadis, chakras, and kundalini

We cannot begin our practice of Babaji's Kriya Yoga without some discussion of the subtle body. Our physical body is made up of *nadis* of channels of energy, which support *prana* in the body. There are five main types of *prana*, different only in their function...*prana, apana, vyana, samana* and *udana*. There are some 72, 000 *nadis* which make up the body but only three that will concern us here and only one has a purely spiritual function: i*da, pingala* and *sushumna*. In everyone the *ida* and *pingala* are active.

As we breathe through the nostrils the *prana* goes in and out through these *nadis*. The *sushumna* however, in most people is not active even though various activities in life would not be possible without the *sushumna*. These three nadis lie inside the spinal column on a subtle level. The *sushumna* is inside the spinal cord and the *ida* is to the left and the *pingala* to the right. The *sushumna* extends from below the base of the spine all the way to the crown of the head. The unfolding of the *sushumna* is the path of liberation.

At the base of the *sushumna* is the *kundalini shakti,* which may be defined as "our potential power and consciousness." It is metaphorically represented as a coiled serpent with its mouth at the entrance to the *sushumna*. The *kundalini* has two aspects, an outer aspect that manifests in worldly existence, which is always functioning to some degree supporting out lives. As Mother Nature, She is the power for all our senses and actions. But She has an inner aspect that must be awakened that will lead us to higher states of consciousness, which are normally lying dormant. Once awakened She transforms us on every level of our being and takes care of our life as well. She releases great creative power.

Along the spine one has seven major psycho-energetic centers known as chakras, located in the axis of the body from the genitals in men, the vagina in women up to the crown of the head. These centers cannot be seen with the naked eye, however they can sometimes be felt and once they are pierced by the awakened *kundalini* they have very definite psychological states associated with them. Normally we are working in the lower three *chakras, muladhara, svadhisthana,* and *manipura,* which are ego-centered and related to survival, sexuality and feelings of pride and will. They relate to the mind and its patterns and preferences. Ideally the energy flowing through these lower chakras will create a strong foundation for the expression of the higher energies of the spirit and our highest potential. When the fourth chakra, the *anahata chakra*, at great spiritual center found at the space of the physical heart is opened, subtle experiences begin to take place and also inner purification. We begin to experience our inner being, and get a sense of our infinite identity. We experience the unconditional love and expansion of the human spirit. Often we experience waves, or thrills of love, which flow through every pore of the body, along with love for the Lord and feelings that needs of others are as important as our own. Sometimes an ability to heal comes with the opening of this chakra. The throat, the *vishuddhi*, is the seat of creativity and truth; when it opens it brings substance to our ideas, and we are able to express ourselves more creatively, truthfully and eloquently. With the opening of the third eye, the *ajna chakra,* the mind becomes one-pointed and thoughts become quieted in deep meditation. We may experience a sense of Intuitive knowing in the form of clairaudience, clairvoyance. Sometimes one is overwhelmed with inner fragrances or celestial sounds, the divine *nada*. Once the crown chakra, the *sahasrara* opens, we open fully to the flow of Intuition. This is the abode of Absolute Reality where one experiences the Presence of the Divine everywhere.

The purifying power of *kundalini*

On her journey to the *sahasrara*, *kundalini* passes through all the sense organs, purifying them and stimulating new strength. As long as the chakras of the sense organs are not purified, the senses work in an ordinary manner, but when they are purified, they acquire divine powers and even the physical senses become sharpened and refined. *Kundalini* is known also as *prana shakti*.

Ayurveda tells us that *prana shakti,* the energy of the universe, is used in the normal functioning of the body as an energy called *retas*. *Retas* or *bindu* is essentially semen, both male (white) and female (red) sexual fluids, which develops in the body naturally and nature utilizes it. Normally excess energy is dissipated or thrown out of the body, unless we practice some discipline of conservation, or some discipline of purity, in order for the energy to continue to increase and gather and converts itself into heat, *tapas*. The movement of *bindu* is closely connected to the breath and to the circulation of the life energy related to pranayama. *Bindu* or *retas* converts into *tapas*, creative heat. Everything that we create comes from *tapas.* The more *tapas* we have the more creative energy we have available.

When the *tapas* is formed in the body there is tremendous increase in vital force, and it is expressed as dynamism. We become more dynamic. By *tapas,* our will-power is activated. If we take care, nourish, cherish and promote the growth of heat without dissipating it, it will turn into *tejas.* *Tejas* is light, brilliance. *Tejas* is reflected as light in the face, a light in the body. T*ejas* has a direct effect on the brain. The brain becomes activated. *Tejas* enhances brain-power and increases memory power.

As both *tapas* and *tejas* are increased they turn into electricity. As electricity courses through the body there is both more dynamic power and intellectual brilliance. The electricity transforms *tejas* into *ojas.* *Ojas* is the primal creative energy of ether. It is very pure. The energy of ether is the purest creative energy on the physical plane. One has the power to create things. With continual purification *ojas* turns into *virya,* which is spiritual power, which facilitates superconscious ecstasy and realization of the Self. This form of life force is the radiance of the Supreme Consciousness, or the Self.

The Practice of Kriya Yoga Sadhana

As a Kriya Yoga sadhak, gradually increase the time you devote to spiritual practices for they are a sure method that will integrate awareness into the very matrix of your everyday life. Asana, pranayama, mantra, and meditation are not goals in themselves, but a means to an end. The combined Kriya practices lead ultimately to the experience of samadhi, cognitive absorption, a breathless state of communion with the Lord. But even before this, the techniques should lead you to become increasingly aware in the "little things of life." All of your experiences thus become a field for your practice of "sadhana." You will begin to see that in every moment that we are present, there is an opportunity for progress to be made. And you will begin to live a life that wants to grow and perfect itself.

7. Imagine

A new year begins. What will it bring? More of the same? Perhaps it need not be so. Imagine yourself creating the life that you were born to realize. Do you now feel trapped in a relationship, a job or locale, which doesn't meet your needs? Everything is amenable to change, if only one can let go of rigid thinking, fears, self-doubts, and negative attitudes.

"But what is it that I should be doing?" you ask. This question brings us close to the reason for our existence, and until and unless we seek an answer to it, we will be like a leaf in the wind, blown about by desires, which constantly invade us from a material culture. What each of must discover is our "dharma," our mission and duties in life. Our ultimate dharma is to realize God, Truth, the Self, "Who Am I?" Books like the "Bhagavad Gita," "Thirumandiram," "Sutras of Patanjali," "Upanishads," may help us to determine the paths we can take to such fulfilment. Along the way to this Self-Realization, however, we meet the results of our past actions, our "karma," which, depending upon how conscious we are, strengthen habitual reactions, or opportunities for us to awaken and to allow the Divine to work through us. Each day, there are many dozens of new situations and events that provide us with a choice. We can react unconsciously according to old mental and emotional patterns, or we can calmly center and attune ourselves to the inspiration available to us if only we listen.

Daily we have the opportunity, in our practice of Kriya Yoga to meet life on a new plateau of self-awareness, and so cultivate continuous bliss. Daily we have the opportunity to dive deep within the very heart of God - Self - Absolute Being, Consciousness and Bliss.

Centered in our hearts, what is it that we are to do?

The answer is to listen to the "tappings" of that Divine "orchestra conductor," who you may like to imagine with the beautiful form of Kriya Babaji Nagaraj. Daily allow your consciousness to soar, to expand, to embrace all, and as you return to the so-called "mundane" world of work, relationships, housekeeping, shopping, hold onto that sacred space you have nurtured during deep meditation. In this sacred space, let go of the sense of being the "doer," and affirm: "not my will, but may Thy will be done." In this sacred space, allow the images and inspiration that come to you, to provide you with your agenda for the coming day's tasks and challenges. Turn to the Master and ask for guidance, then listen. As you allow your imagination to develop, it will develop your inspiration, and the guidance and resources you need to fulfil your earthly mission will arrive "just at the right time." Play your part, always listening to the rhythm being established by your Satguru.

8. Getting It and Keeping It

We are engaged, individually and as a group in getting and keeping Self Realization. There are times, perhaps when engaged in our practice, or even spontaneously, when the Self evident truth of the Absolute Reality, "*sat chit ananda*," absolute Being, Consciousness, and Bliss dawns upon us. At such times when we center our consciousness on the subject "I AM;" it shines, or comes to the foreground, and our experience, whether it be on the physical, emotional, mental or intellectual planes fades into the background and becomes the object. When we identify with who we truly are, and not with the phantasmagoria of our experiences, we are One. There is not even an iota of doubt about it. There is only effulgent self-awareness, which sees only its Self everywhere. At such times, there is no gap between where we are and where we want to be. Desires subside. The mind calms. There is nothing more to do, to learn, to become. Bliss is.

However, at other times, this Self awareness fades into the background, as we allow the mind to move in its habitual patterns of identifying with what it is not: its worries, desires, sense experiences, and various emotions, and thoughts. We may tell ourselves that we want Self-realization but instead, we allow ourselves to identify with the object of experience and not with consciousness itself. So many people become initiated in a spiritual system of practices and then wonder why they have not yet realized God? They expect that simply by learning to use the tools offered by yoga, they will realize their aspirations.

While the tools and the aspirations may remain, however faded, what is missing is the will to apply oneself moment to moment. It is not what you did last year, or what you intend to do later on that is important in the field of yoga and Self-realization, but what are you doing in each moment. You can choose to bring awareness into every act, into every mundane moment of the day or you can allow your old habits of distraction, inertia and unconsciousness dominate your life.

Yogic sadhana is reminding you constantly to center and be aware. To identify with the "I AM," and to see your experience as a passing show, without identifying with it or becoming attached to it. Whether it is postures, pranayama, meditation, mantras or bhakti yoga, or jnana or karma yoga, the purpose is the same. To remind and to train your consciousness to remain pure and free, until it becomes spontaneous and effortless. Because of the habits of the mind, this requires effort for a long time. One should expect failures, but consider them as stepping stones to success. "If you do not give up, you are bound to attain the goal one day" was an often repeated teaching of my teacher.

Ultimately, yogic sadhana has as its purpose to know without a doubt the answer to the following questions. "Who Am I?" or "Who worries?" or "Who feels this emotion?" or "Who is it that is reacting so?" You will know the answer when you perceive by the light of consciousness the pure, undisturbed essence of our being, the "I AM," as distinct from the thoughts, emotions and experiences which may currently dominate . This pure Self is met easily every night during deep sleep. Who does not look forward to meeting his or her self during sleep? It is a universal time of rejoicing. A deep sleep is so blissful. This bliss is experienced also in deep meditation or whenever one succeeds in being centered in the awareness of the moment.

Getting and keeping Self-realization is a matter of making it our moment to moment priority. There is no time to procrastinate. Make every moment in your life count, as though it were your last. Make every event, however mundane or insignificant, an opportunity to center and to practice self-awareness. Notice how old habits try to distract or overwhelm your self-awareness. Monitor your breath: it will indicate to you when you are no longer present. God is not far-away, it is you who are mostly absent, lost in your dreams. Celebrate the Presence by being present. Know that there is only One Absolute Being permeating your whole universe. Be aware and so be in bliss.

9. The Art of Meditation, You and What You Are Not

The practice of meditation is becoming more and more popular. Yet it remains widely misunderstood, even by those who claim to practice it. If you tell someone that you "meditate" they are likely to ask: "Oh, are you trying to make your mind go blank?" If that is all that meditation is, one might suggest that meditation is simply an unconscious state. Others may even fear meditation, out of ignorance of what it is and what it can do for them. We often fear what we do not understand. In writing this article, I hope to provide some understanding of the process of meditation, its immense benefits and how to get started.

Why has meditation become popular in recent decades?

Meditation has become popular in recent decades for several reasons:

1. many scientific studies have proven it to be effective in control-
    ling the effects of stress, reversing heart disease, reducing blood
    pressure and in promoting emotional well being. Consequently,
    doctors recommend it to patients who are suffering from these
    conditions.

2. a growing interest in spirituality. Many persons who go to church,
    for example are no longer satisfied with merely having an intel-
    lectual or emotional experience there. They want a spiritual ex-
    perience as well. Spirituality, as distinct from religion, empha-
    sizes that which is formless, and this can be experienced when the
    mind becomes quiet. Meditation is one means for quieting the
    mind.

3. a growing dissatisfaction with the religious approaches to the
    great questions of life: why do bad things happen to good peo-
    ple? Why am I suffering? Is there a God? As people become more
    independent in their thinking, they aspire to find the truth of
    things for themselves, without being limited by dogma or the be-
    lief systems of religious institutions.

4. a large number of books and the arrival of teachers of meditation,
    particularly from Asia, where meditation has a long history and
    refined development, has made meditation much more accessible.
    One no longer has to enter a monastery to learn it. The examples
    of spiritual masters have inspired many to seek "Self-realization,"
    as the goal of life.

What is meditation?

I like to define meditation as "being continually aware of a chosen object or subject." Therefore, meditation allows you to be who you really
are, because your higher nature, which is pure consciousness, is always
meditating, always aware. The difficulty arises with the fact that you
rarely adopt the perspective of your higher nature, that of your soul, that
of a witnessing consciousness, if you like. You are in the habit of allowing your consciousness to become completely absorbed in the experiences that arise within your mind, prompted by what comes through your
five senses, memories or emotions. Or, you are dispersed in many directions. It is your lower human nature, which causes your mind to become

absorbed in such things, just like when you are absorbed in a book, movie or television program. Meditation is a process of training your mind to "let go" of what it is normally identified with, so that you can remember to be who you really are. In other words, meditation allows you "to get in touch with your self."

All schools of meditation agree on the above definition of meditation. Seeking to become "continually aware" is the goal of all schools. What distinguishes different schools from one another, is the object or subject that is chosen, in order to train the mind to "let go" of its ordinary preoccupations. Many schools choose the breath, and simply follow it, without trying to control it. Other schools recommend a mantra, one or more syllables, which when repeated, induce a higher state of awareness. Other schools focus on a visualized form, like a mandala (a geometric form representing the macrocosm in the microcosm, or the universe within the human body), which serves to center the mind, and to neutralize its tendency to wander. Still others cultivate a train of thoughts related to an abstract subject, such as love, truth, beauty, suffering, or destiny.

Depending upon the goal of the particular practice, the technique may vary. Many schools of meditation seek to quiet the mind in order to transcend it, to seek the deepest peace and tranquility within. In the tradition of Babaji's Kriya Yoga, meditation is defined as "the scientific art of mastering the mind." This is implies a broad agenda with many more objectives, because the mind has many levels and functions, and potential faculties yet to be developed. It includes techniques of meditation to cleanse the subconscious of habitual tendencies that are the source of much suffering. Other techniques are used to develop one's power of concentration, something needed to succeed in all areas of life. Still others develop the intellect and its conceptual power, along with opening one to great insight and intuitive power. Still others encourage one to become a co-creator in one's own life experiences, developing the intuitive, the psychic and the superconscious levels of consciousness. For this reason there are a large number of meditation techniques taught in Babaji's Kriya Yoga. Each technique is like a specialized tool that one may use for different purposes.

The obstacles to meditation

Meditation is a science and an art. When practiced correctly, it will create the same results and benefits for any and all practitioners. If it was only a science, however, meditation would yield it promised results as soon as you have understood the method and tried it. Unfortunately, the tendencies of your lower nature, distraction, laziness, restlessness, boredom or sleep will resist meditation. Meditation requires that you change your habitual physical and mental tendencies, and so meditation is also an art. As in any art, meditation requires diligent practice for a long time to develop the skill to overcome the habits and human nature which resist change. It is through your often-repeated thoughts, words and actions that habits are established. When these habits involve desires or fears, then you become driven by such, and lose awareness of your higher self, that of your soul, the spiritual dimension of your being wherein pure consciousness or awareness resides. Meditation allows you to access your thoughts, words and actions, even before they happen.

The nine obstacles to continuous inner awareness are:

1. Disease. It is both physical and mental. It results from how we react to the stress of life. What happens when you are sick? Your mind becomes distracted by its symptoms: the discomfort, the pain, the fatigue. You are absorbed by it. If I ask you "are you sick?" your response is "I am sick." You are not sick. Your body is! So, to avoid becoming absorbed by it, watch yourself. Be a witness to the illness. Of course, an ounce of prevention is worth a pound of cure, so cultivate healthy living habits so that you do not fall sick. Develop a balance in your diet, in exercise, relaxation and rest. Similarly, avoid emotional disease by learning to "let go" of difficult emotions in daily life. Mental disease involves worry, fear and obsession. While everyone may experience passing thoughts of this type, a healthy mind will not cultivate them, but learn to let them go. Reserve your mental energy for the problems at hand. Detach from negative thinking. Cultivate positive thoughts, auto-suggestion and affirmations to replace negative thinking. Avoid negative activities and persons who may feed negative mental habits. Such things as anger, worry, fear, complaining are examples of things to avoid. By not indulging in negative thinking such habits will gradually weaken.

2. Dullness. Dullness occurs when there is inadequate energy to maintain continuous awareness. Until Self-realization is established firmly, it requires effort to keep part of our consciousness standing back as a witness. This effort requires a minimum amount of energy. So we must avoid getting ourselves so fatigued by overwork, or lack of sleep that we lose the perspective of the witness of our thoughts, words and deeds. Like the

means to overcoming disease, we need to cultivate healthy, balanced living habits to keep our energy high, and to avoid energy robbing activities such as intoxicants, excessive indulgence in talking, eating, watching television and too much work. We may need to simplify our life and let go of unnecessary activities or responsibilities.

3. Doubt is the tendency of the mind to question, and when it is not accompanied by a seeking for answers, it may leave one cynical and unprepared to continue to make efforts. This is particularly a problem among persons who are overly intellectual. Even when they have been given a satisfactory answer, their intellect enjoys doubting for the sake of doubting. Their intellect gets so much satisfaction from the game of questioning and seeking new sources of stimulus. Doubts can help one to ask good questions, but often one needs to be patient before one can find the answer. So, write down your doubts in the form of clear questions in your notebook, and seek opportunities to find their answers from your teachers, sacred texts, or during meditation.

There are some questions which can only be answered when one changes perspective. For example, one can never "know" God. One can never know what is "consciousness" either. For "knowing" implies the separate existence of the knower, known and their relationship in knowing. Where does God and consciousness not exist? If they are indeed everywhere, there is no possibility of knowing them as something other than one Self. By changing perspective, however, being completely present, and identified with the essence of One Self, the one can become conscious of God, and conscious of what is conscious. One can realize that while the body or mind may suffer, "I" am not the body or the mind, and that the purpose of suffering is to help us to realize this.

4. Carelessness is inattention, dispersion, a habitual lack of focus. In our fast paced modern lifestyle, many persons feel obligated to try to do more than one thing at a time, and so become careless. Their consciousness is absorbed in many tasks at once, and if not, they seek multiple distractions, for example from the radio or television, even while eating or driving. They assume that the more they can do, or the more they can take in through their five senses, the happier they will be. The truth is just the opposite. By being present with whatever you are doing, joy arises spontaneously. When you are not present, you confuse happiness with the presence or absence of something outside of yourself. One can overcome

the habit of carelessness by learning to focus the attention on one thing at a time, and being a witness to oneself while doing it.

5. Laziness is a habit, due to discouragement, lack of enthusiasm or inspiration. It is essentially an emotional state, and as such is subject to our conscious will. It is not due to fatigue to dullness, which can be corrected by rest and healthy living habits. Ask yourself, when you feel lazy or discouraged, "could I let this go." Cultivate positive emotional states through the devotional activities such as singing; or use auto-suggestions to counter negative feelings. We can also overcome this habit by gradually replacing it with positive habits such as regularity in our practice, reading inspirational literature, association with persons who will inspire and feed us emotionally and mentally. Keep a record of how you use your time, and eliminate those activities which cause you to feel discouraged, like too much television, to much work, not sufficient physical exercise which will stimulate the endorphins, and which make you feel enthusiastic.

6. Sensuality occurs where desires are not detached from but rather encouraged. It is fantasizing about the object of desire, rather than the actual experience of the object.   You begin to feel that "unless I can eat that particular food, or drink, or be with that person, or engage in that particular desire, I will not be happy." It is human to have desires, but as you become more aware, you can detach from them, you can refuse to continue to entertain thoughts of lust, greed, and hunger. By indulging such thoughts you deny the reality of your true source of happiness: the inner Being, Consciousness, Bliss. Today, in our modern, materialistic culture, we are constantly bombarded with the message "indulge" yourself in this fantasy. Advertising tries to convince us that if we only consume or own this product we will be fulfilled. The reality, is sadly the opposite.

This is not to say that you should avoid sensual activity. There is nothing inherently wrong in eating, drinking, feeling things with your skin, or consuming or owning any material object. Sensuality is fantasizing about how good you will feel, or how happy you will be when you have that experience or material thing. It is a confusion of the mind, based upon our fundamental ignorance wherein we confuse the source of our happiness with something outside of ourselves. So, whenever you are enjoying something through the five senses, do enjoy it fully, by being a witness to it. When fantasies come however, detach from them. Be present with whatever you are experiencing at that moment.

7. False perception is not seeing the underlying reality. It is due to fundamental ignorance of who we are. Because of egoism, we confuse the subject, "I am" with the objects of our experience. We confuse the permanent with the impermanent. So, the mind is constantly distracted by the objects of experience through the five senses, and our consciousness is totally absorbed in the passing show. It is like someone who goes to the movie theater and becomes completely absorbed in the film until the end. They forget who they are. That person ignores the one permanent constant: the light of the projector and the screen on which the lighted images are playing. By cultivating presence, taking one moment at a time, we can overcome this "false perception." We can easily perceive that which always is, within and without. When you feel yourself getting caught up in the drama of life, in the "film," take a deep breath, and be a witness to what is, right there and then. To break the habit of false perception, reserve a part of your day for meditation, and a part of your vacation time for retreats. Gradually, the problem of false perception will diminish.

8. Failure to reach firm ground occurs when there is a lack of patience and perseverance. So often, students of Yoga, particularly in the West, expect instant coffee, instant tea, and instant Self-realization. They are not prepared to work intensively and for a long time to bring it about. They have cultivated expectations that it will be easy and come soon, and easily become impatient when their own resistance becomes obvious. Usually, they flit from one teacher to another, always looking for someone to do it for them. They do not take responsibility for their own bad habits. The thing that most distinguishes those who succeed in becoming enlightened from those who do not is "patience." When you fall down, or fail to act as you would have wanted, rather than indulging feelings of inadequacy or discouragement or impatience, treat your failures as stepping stones to success. Cultivate a routine of practice and gradually increase the amount of time you allocate to your practice. Tackle your small bad habits first. Overcome them with auto-suggestion and detachment, this will give you the confidence to overcome deep seated habits.

9. Instability is the mental or emotional state which occurs when there is a failure to maintain a calm equilibrium during the highs and lows of life. It occurs when there is a lack of consistency in one's practice. One becomes lost in the transitory show of life. This shows up, for example, when one becomes·elated when things go well, and disappointed or angry

or frustrated when things go badly. One's happiness depends upon success, not failure, gain not loss, praise, not blame, etc. However, all dualities are inherently unstable, and try as we might to hold onto things, they are very fragile. Why put one's faith in something which is going to pass? To avoid "instability" cultivate equanimity in the face of the various dualities, as described above. Notice the sense of well being that it is possible to have within oneself, despite what your karma may bring to your doorstep that day. Lighten up. Don't worry, but be present, and so happy. When difficulties come, take a deep breath if you find your mind or body starting to react in their habitual negative ways with expressions of anger or frustration. Remember, "this too shall pass." Remember this also when things go well.

These nine obstacles to continuous awareness, the goal of meditation, are mentioned in Patanjali's Yoga Sutras I.30. While the study of such classic texts is an aid, there is no substitute for regular diligent practice. There is no higher authority than your own experience. So, go ahead and enjoy the new, higher consciousness which comes as you begin to implement the above recommendations for meditation. Begin now, and make each moment count, living fully in the present.

How to get started?

"We are dreaming with our eyes open" is a saying of the Yoga Siddhas, the supreme masters of yoga. This saying characterizes the fundamental dilemma of human existence. We are "dreaming" whenever we are absorbed in the movements of the mind: sense perceptions, conceptualizations, fantasies, memories and sleep, according to the Siddha Patanjali in his Yoga Sutras. This incisive diagnosis called for a prescription, and the Siddhas responded with the development of many techniques to wake us up from our dream state. Patanjali prescribes twelve different methods of meditation to calm the mind. Depending upon one's particular nature one method may be more effective than others. Some experimentation with different methods is therefore recommended, to help determine which works best for you.

Meditation is not really something that you do! It is truly who you are! It cannot be divorced from the rest of your life. So, learning to meditate begins with some preparation so that how you live your life does not overwhelm your attempts at meditation. Meditation begins with being present, and this requires several things. When you are present you are giving your undivided attention to what is happening right now. As we are conditioned by life's experiences to dwell on the past or to be apprehensive about the future, some preparation is required to de-condition the ordinary habit driven mind. Formal meditation training in the Eastern schools such as Classical Yoga includes several phases. One of the most well known is the eight limbed (*astanga*) or steps:

1. *yamas*, or five restraints, which will optimize social relationships and ensure that they do not become a source of mental disturbance. These are five: avoiding any words or actions, even thoughts which might harm others; speaking only what is truthful; seeing others as spiritual beings first and not as sex objects; avoiding taking what does not belong to you; avoiding greed.

2. *niyamas*, or five observances: cultivating pure loving thoughts, words and actions; contentment, being grateful for what one has; continuous practice of remembrance of our higher self, and letting go of false identification with the mind's movements; self-study: through study of sacred texts and such things as recording in a journal one's meditations; turning continuously towards the Divine with love and reverence for all of its manifestations.

3. *asana*, the practice of yoga postures to produce stability and relaxation;

4. *pranayama,* the practice of special breathing exercises to calm the mind and to access one's potential power and consciousness

5. *pratyahara*, withdrawal of one's consciousness from the senses, avoidance of mental dispersion in many unnecessary activities.

6. *dharana*, developing one's power of concentration on a single object.

7. *dhyana,* or meditation proper, as defined above, developing continuous awareness, with whatever object or experience.

8. The above leads to the ultimate goal of meditation, referred to as *samadhi*, or cognitive absorption, in which one transcends the ordinary ego perspective of being separate from objects of experience; one becomes Self realized.

By recognizing that so many things including our body and its health, our mental and emotional habits, our social relationships all have an effect on our ability to meditate, one will derive the maximum benefit and avoid many of the pitfalls that beginning meditators experience. So it is recommended that in addition to learning and experimenting with various simple meditations, one begin to observe the first five phases of ashtanga yoga, mentioned above.

In particular, just before sitting for meditation, the beginning student will find that the practice of some yoga postures and breathing exercises will energize and relax the body-mind complex, and help one to avoid sleep, a common source of difficulty.

Posture for sitting

The best posture for sitting is the one you feel most comfortable in. So, experiment with different positions. If your knees are tight and you find it difficult to sit on the floor cross legged, sit on the edge of a chair, with your back erect in its natural "S" curve, and your hand resting on your knees or joined with the palms turned upwards. After doing the yoga postures, which open your hips, strengthen your knees and develop a strong and flexible spine, you will be able to sit or kneel on the floor with or without the support of a cushion or small bench. There are many types, and so experiment with them and find the one that supports you most comfortably.

Breathing

There is great benefit to take some long deep breaths before you begin your meditation. It can be beneficial to count your breaths, counting how long it takes to inhale and to exhale and then to try to lengthen your exhalation to be twice as long, as your inhalation. For instance if you breathe in for a count of 6 seconds, breathe out for a count of 12 seconds. The inhalation is connected to the sympathetic nervous system, which governs the "fight or flight" response; the exhalation is connected to the parasympathetic nervous system, which governs the relaxation response. By emphasizing the exhalation, you begin to relax the body and the mind, enabling you to enter the meditative perspective.

Beginning meditation techniques

As described above, there are many different techniques, and they vary according to their purpose.

1. Hamsa

Breathe deeply several times. As you breathe in, feel yourself filling up with energy. As you breathe out feel yourself letting go of the tension and fatigue.

Now relax into your normal breathing patterns and and begin to repeat the word "I," followed by a pause. Each time you say "I," notice what you become aware of. Perhaps at first, there are physical sensations. Then perhaps some thoughts or emotions. Each time you say "I" imagine its like adjusting the lens of a microscope and you're beneath the microscope. At some point you notice that all these sensations, thoughts, and emotions are appearing and disappearing on a kind of screen; like the images of a television screen. Then you notice the screen is made up of light particles. As you go deeper and deeper within with the word "I," you notice that these particles are moving. Particles of light everywhere, inside you, around you, moving through you. At this level it becomes difficult to distinguish where you end and other things begin. The space is widening between the particles.

If I ask you now, who are you, what would you say? It's no longer adequate to refer to your name or some memory or some sensation. Here, like the mystic, you can say I Am That. I am That infinite being from which everything comes and to which everything returns. I am like a vast ocean out of which so many waves appear on the surface. Up until now you've been living only on the surface of your being. Your consciousness has been focused on the individual waves, thoughts, feelings, and emotions. Now your consciousness has expanded and you're aware of that ocean of being that transcends you, that supports you, that contains you, which is infinite and eternal. "I Am That," says the mystic. I was never born. That which I truly am has always existed. Everything is within me. I am in everything. Everything comes and everything goes…thoughts, sensations, emotions…but I remain, the one constant throughout all of the events and dramas of my life. Becoming aware of this one constant, its reality is beyond any doubt. It is self-evident.

How do you maintain this perspective? Your breath is always naturally reminding you of the truth of this perspective. The breath gives you a natural reminder. Each inhalation it whispers a sound like "ham," which means in sanskrit "I Am." During exhalation it makes a sound like "sa," which in sanskrit means "That." Whenever you notice the inhalation, mentally say "ham" and remember "I Am." Whenever you notice the exhalation, mentally say "sa" and remember "That." Make no effort to control the breath, simply follow it. If other thoughts come, do not try to chase them away. Just return to "ham-sa." Gradually as your breathing slows down, the thoughts will become quieter. This subtly emphasizes the subjective side of absolute reality. I Am. If you reverse it, it emphasizes the objective side of reality: That, I Am. Two sides of one coin. I am that I am. So for at least ten minutes be very calm, focus on your breath and repeat "ham" as you breathe in and "sa" as you breathe out. And remember, I Am That....

2. Japa or the repetition of a mantra

Repeat continuously, aloud or mentally a thought such as "I AM" or "Peace," or "It's all Divine Mother Nature" or "Om, Om, Om," (the sound of universal energy, which exists in everything as a vibration or sound), "Amen," or "Tat Twam Asi" (That I am). This practice is known as *japa*, the continuous repetition of mantras. They remind one that all is One, and that everything is only apparent. This allows you to bring a third person perspective into whatever you happen to be doing at the time. There is you digging the ditch, and there is the ditch which is being dug, but there is also third party, one which is disinterested, but which regards it all with total love and appreciation for how it all is. In so doing you can transcend the ordinary egoistic perspective of "I am digging" the ditch, and begin to cultivate the perspective of a witness.

3. Tratak

Set a candle at a distance of about twenty inches from you face. The height of the flame should be level with your eyes. Sit up straight with your spine erect. With your eyes open, gaze at the flame, blinking freely whenever they feel too dry. Start with five minutes, and gradually increase the time. Allow thoughts to come and to go, and avoid trying to do anything. Just be with the flame until you and flame become one. You may repeat a mantra simultaneously if you wish.

The above exercises numbered one to three, are formal meditations done with the eyes closed, but this one, Tradak, is done only with the eyes open. They all help one to prepare oneself for meditation in daily life, which is described next.

4. Witnessing

There are hundreds of you's, each a different part of your personality. There is the angry you, the sad you, the nervous you, the proud you, the hurt you, and the lustful you, just to name a few. Anyone of them can make a mistake for which the rest of you may pay a heavy price for many years. But they come and go. There is one You however, which is always there behind all of the others. It is called the Witness. It is not doing anything. It witnesses everything get done. It is not thinking. It is watching thoughts come and go. It is not feeling any emotion. It is watching the emotions arise and fall. It can be done with eyes closed in formal meditation posture, or during activities, initially routine ones.

You may adopt the perspective of the witness initially by slowing down, perhaps taking a few deep breaths, and watch yourself do whatever you are doing. Initially you are seeking to develop calmness. Calmness is not the absence of thoughts, but being present with the thoughts. The substance of consciousness remains undisturbed, and thoughts, sensations or emotions pass by, like a flock of birds in the sky, leaving the sky undisturbed.

You watch yourself walking, eating, picking up and arranging things. Then the phone rings, and you pick it up and begin talking. At that point you forget to be the witness because some other "you" jumps into the foreground. Only much later do you remember that you were attempting to be the witness. You resolve not to forget, and try again. But many subtle "you's" continue to distract you from your resolve. After awhile you begin to notice that while you still forget often, you remember sooner. Falling asleep begins to set off an alarm which wakes up again. This is a important stage in the development of the witness, as it is beginning to become automatic.

When you continue with the practice, you begin to notice some difficult emotions arising, but before they do, you are able to let go of them, because you are the witness.

As you begin to live more calmly as the witness, breaking identification with the many old "you's," you begin to recognize how the laws of the universe are operating, from a deep intuitive perspective. Bliss ensues whenever you remain in the Witness perspective, even though life may be difficult. The perspective of separation, as the Witness, at some point begins to end. While you have used this dualistic perspective, it is transcended as You the Seer, and everything else, the Seen, is transcended. What remains is the One. Silence rules the mind. Into it great insights may then descend from one's higher intelligence.

Patience and perseverance

A beginner may only really meditate for ten percent of a session, because ninety percent of the session, the mind is wandering or falling asleep, or distracted by the body. With practice however, meditation becomes more and more continuous. As with any art, one needs to persevere and be patient with one's self. The practice requires attention and skill and these develop slowly. You can accelerate your development if you practice every day at the same time, preferably at least twice a day. By devising strategies to prevent the following nine obstacles to continuous awareness in daily life you will also make rapid progress in "mastering of the mind."

10. By Contentment, Supreme Joy is Attained

What has "contentment" to do with the practice of Yoga? Patanjali who compiled one of the first texts on the subject of Yoga, lays out some preliminary practices, prior to the practice of his "Kriya Yoga". These preliminary practices he refers to as the "eight-limbed" or "*ashtanga yoga*" in Sutra II.29: "The eight limbs of Yoga" are: 1. yama (restraint), 2. niyama (observance), 3. asana, (posture), 4. pranayama (breath control), 5. pratyahara (sense withdrawal), 6. dharana (concentration), 7. dhyana (meditation), 8. samadhi (cognitive absorption).

The yamas or restraints are non-violence, truthfulness, non-stealing, chastity and greedlessness. The niyamas or observances consist of purity, contentment, accepting but not causing pain, self-study and surrender to the Lord. In contemporary schools of yoga, the emphasis is upon the yoga postures, and the yamas and niyamas are usually ignored. Perhaps it is out of an unwillingness to engage the moral principles which they imply. Or perhaps it is because in our contemporary materialistic culture, they strike one as being counter-cultural. However, without understanding our cultural blinders, our efforts to practice yoga are likely to be frustrated repeatedly.

Defining the niyama of "contentment," in Sutra II.42, Patanjali tells us: "By contentment, supreme joy is gained." Contentment (*samtosha*), involves neither liking nor disliking; it occurs when one is simply being oneself. The nature of our being is absolute joy (ananda). There is nothing to do, but to appreciate, or observe it.

Contentment is an inner poise, which implies harmony, delight in oneself and inner love, wherein one is untroubled by difficulties around oneself. Whether anyone feels it, or not, is due to his or her openness to it. It arises spontaneously when we practice "nityananada kriya," taught in the second initiation of Babaji's Kriya Yoga.

The problem is that because of our cultural conditioning, we forget to cultivate contentment! It is as if we are programmed to believe that by suffering, we will eventually become happy!

A videocassette entitled "Affluenza," which one of our students recently gave to me, speaks of the spiritual emptiness, physical and mental disease and environmental disasters being caused by our "consumer society." It also speaks hopefully of the 20 percent of North Americans who are now a part of a movement towards "voluntary simplicity."

Paul Ray in his book, "Cultural Creatives" documents how nearly 50 million of North Americans, are becoming "cultural creatives," people who care deeply about saving the planet, nurturing relationships, expressing peace, embodying social justice, and cultivating authenticity, self-actualization, spirituality and self-expression.

Recently, 320 American Buddhist leaders met in Northern California to discuss among other things the difficulty of reconciling American culture, with its emphasis on free-market capitalism, greed, competition and envy of material things with Buddhism, with its emphasis on transcendence of greed, envy and the pursuit of material goods. The Dalai Lama urged a return to basics: the cultivation of compassion and freedom from anger and greed. The problem, as pointed out by one participant, is not with money itself, but with the role that money plays in the psyche and life of the person.

Discontent, is of course the opposite of contentment. It is also what drives our modern materialistic culture, as expressed in our competitiveness, our seeking of status, our need to possess more, do more and know more. Even contemporary "personal growth" seminars, too often feed this discontent by promising us prosperity or experiences, if we will simply attend!

Greedlessness (*aparigrahah*) includes not fantasizing over material possessions, nor coveting things belonging to others. Often people fantasize that if they could only become suddenly rich, by winning the lottery or marrying someone with lots of money, or winning big in the stock market, they would find lasting happiness. This is pure folly. Indulging in such fantasy simply distracts one from the inner source of lasting joy.

How can each of us overcome these tendencies which the consumer culture has left deeply engrained within our minds, and be content? In sutra II.33, Patanjali offers to us a solution: "When bound by negative thoughts, their opposite (i.e. positive) ones should be cultivated. (This is) *pratipaksa bhavanam.*" Rather than indulging or rationalizing them, Patanjali prescribes direct action: the cultivation of opposite thoughts. For example, if we envy, we can summons feelings of gratitude and contentment for what we already possess. While Patanjali does not elaborate upon this practice, we know that siddhas like him were first-rate psychologists. To counter deep-seated tendencies towards negative thinking required regular and diligent practice of such things as affirmations, autosuggestion and self-hypnosis. The subconscious mind, not unlike a computer, continues to operate according to suggestions which are programmed into it since early childhood even when they are harmful or cause suffering. Such suggestions come from our parents, teachers, friends, the mass media, cultural symbols and values. It is a wonder that our teachers and authorities have for the most part failed to emphasize or teach the scientific art of auto-suggestion and affirmation indicated by Patanjali in this verse.

Too often, those who enter a spiritual lifestyle assume that their spiritual practices will automatically heal deep-seated psychological conflicts. While psychotherapy may initially help, it often lacks a wider spiritual perspective. Ultimately the healing process requires each person to skilfully counter all unwholesome thoughts and emotions without merely suppressing them. The practice of detachment will help us all to cultivate contentment in daily life, leading us to, Patanjali promises us, "supreme joy."

11. A Man's Home is His Ashram

As we awaken to the spiritual dimension of life, we may find ourselves almost always confronted by a mind which causes us much distraction. This universal human dilemma, wherein our consciousness is completely absorbed in the fluctuations of the mind, the "*vrittis*," such as memories, sense perceptions, sleep, conceptualizations and misconceptions, has been analyzed by Patanjali at the beginning of his Yoga-Sutras (verses (I.5-11). But Patanjali also describes the goal of Yoga, Self-realization throughout his famous text by clearly distinguishing these fluctuations of the mind (the Seen) from the Seer, or the Self. He writes: "Then the Seer abides in his own true form," (verse 1.3) But in the following verse he clearly indicates how prone we are to lose this Self-realization: "Otherwise, there is an identification (of the individuated self) with the fluctuations (of consciousness)." How can we overcome this fundamental ignorance, *avidya* wherein we confuse the Self with the non-Self, the Seer with the Seen, the permanent with the impermanent? Is our Yoga today helping us to remain awake, or making us fall asleep?

Yoga today has become a big business. A recent article in the Yoga Journal estimates that there are over 18 million Americans now practicing some form of Yoga, and that on average they spend $1,500 per year. That adds up to a $27 billion dollar a year industry, only a little bit less than what Microsoft generates each year! Consumer and Corporate America, the yin and the yang of our materialistic culture, has hijacked Yoga.

Is this consumer element of American Yoga creating delusion? Being consumers, driven by a culture and economic system which constantly tells us that the more we consume, the happier we will be, we usually find ourselves "consuming" in the spiritual marketplace: classes in Yoga studios, seminars, cassettes, props, books, teachers, teachings. Always looking outside ourselves for things that will give us what we are missing. For example, most persons who go to Yoga studios do not even practice Yoga at home! They try to get something they feel they are missing from someone else. And far too many of the thousands of Yoga studios that have sprouted up in the shopping malls of America, the great temples of materialism, are promoting this delusion! Make no mistake, there is a great cultural battle going on here. While such goods and services may make us feel or look better, or improve our health, and at best even remind us of our spiritual path, they can only take us a little way towards the goal of authentic Yoga: Self-realization.

Self-realization, wherein one realizes oneself as the Seer, as distinct from the Seen, the experiences, may come in a flash of insight. But Self-realization or *Samadhi* (cognitive absorption) as described by Patanjali in the Sutras 1.40-51 is elusive, as long as we continue to identify with our mind, that is all of the fluctuations, the *vritti* arising within consciousness: the thoughts, sense experiences and memories. At the very beginning of the Yoga-Sutras, in verse I.2, Patanjali tells us that "Yoga is the cessation (of identifying with) the fluctuations (arising within) consciousness." After analyzing these fluctuations he recommends as a solution not a specific method but: "By constant practice and detachment (arises) the cessation (of identifying with the fluctuations of consciousness)." (verse I.12)

But how long will it take? Because of our conditioning, we all want to find the quickest and easiest path. And we are willing to spend for it! But Patanjali tells us in effect that the only currency with any value in the field of Yoga is sincerity: "Thus, the characteristic difference (as to how quickly cognitive absorption is reached depends on whether the yogin's practice is weak, moderate or intense." (verse I.22)

A mild practice is uneven, sporadic, full of doubts, ups and downs and full of distractions, which carry one away. A moderate practice has periods of intensity and devotion, alternating with periods of forgetfulness, distractions and indulgences in negative thinking and habits. An intense practice is characterized by the constant determination to remember the Self and to maintain equanimity through success, and failure, pleasure and pain, growing in love, confidence, patience and sympathy for others. No matter what the intensity of the events or circumstances, no matter how great the play of the illusion filled drama, we continue to see Divinity throughout.

We may often hear our mind making excuses like, "I don't have time to practice Yoga, I have to go to work" or "I wish I had more time to practice." We may also find our mind yearning for a time and place which would be more ideal: "When I retire, I will go to India and live in an ashram." Or "Next year, I am going to go on a retreat at that ashram in the mountains." This of course is just more of the same habitual reaction of the mind, seeking something outside, involved in the duality of the moment such as liking or disliking, success or failure or loss or gain. And as long as we consider our practice of Yoga to be something which we consume, or consume "out there," we will only be reinforcing the mind's game.

You are not the mind. You have a mind. You are Being-Consciousness-Bliss, *Satchitananda*. And in order to fully realize this, in every moment, you must play the game of consciousness: constant Self-awareness. In Babaji's Kriya Yoga, many techniques or *kriyas* are taught to enable one to cultivate awareness in every moment and at all levels of existence, including the *asanas* for the physical, *pranayama* breathing for the vital, *dhyana* meditation for the mental, *mantras* for the intellectual and devotional *bhakti Yoga* for the spiritual dimension of our being. This brings about an integral development and ultimately perfection or *siddhi* at all levels, not merely a spiritual or vertical ascent.

When and how will you do this? As often as you can remember to do so! It is up to you! All Yogic *sadhana* or practices may be summarized as: "everything you do to remember who you are, and everything you do to let go of what you are not." You are probably reading this at home at this very moment. As you read these lines, can you allow part of your consciousness to stand back as a witness, watching your mind read these words? Can you continue to allow your consciousness to be divided into two parts: one part absorbed in seeing, hearing, doing, thinking, feeling and another part simply being aware of everything going on? If so, you will find bliss in each moment. You win this "bliss" whenever you are aware. This "game of consciousness" is the only game worth playing. Every time you remember to play it, you win, every time you forget to be the witness, you suffer, and lose. Even if your karma is delivering roses, and not rotten tomatoes to your doorstep, if you are absorbed by the drama, your mind will soon start worrying about when it will end, and so suffer.

So make your home a place where you will practice this Yogic sadhana in every moment. What do we do at home? Eat, sleep, wash up, relax, play and do housework. Make all of these activities fields of consciousness, opportunities to practice awareness as taught in Babaji's Kriya Yoga. Here are some specific suggestions in each of these areas:

1. Mealtime: when you sit down for a meal, make it a sacred activity, starting from the time you begin the meal preparation. Sing devotional songs or chant mantras, and cultivate the witness as you chop, cook, serve. When you sit down, say a prayer or chant the food dedication mantra: *Ahm Hreem Kram Swahaa, Chitrya Chitra guptraya yamarupy dryah Om Tat Sat Om Kriya Babaji Nama Aum.* Chew each mouth full, practicing being the witness to everything experienced. Even when you are washing the dishes and taking out the garbage, continue to cultivate this Self-awareness.

2. Housework and bill paying. The old dictum, "cleanliness is next to Godliness" applies here too. Maintain your home as though you are expecting God to visit you at any time. By creating a space of order, brightness and cleanliness you will experience more equanimity within yourself. Cultivate the witness as you go about this activity. By learning to budget your expenses according to your revenue, and paying them on time, you will avoid much stress and so free the mind from disturbing reactions.

3. Exercise, bathe and dressing times. Train your mind to focus inwardly as you go about the daily rituals of your Yoga postures practice, your bath and dressing time. Do one thing at a time, with part of your consciousness withdrawn from involvement in the play of the senses and the mind.

4. Playing with your children. Your children can teach how to regain spontaneity, laughter, and being in the present. Seek out opportunities to share with them what you love about life, and encourage them to express themselves. Be a good listener not only to them, but to your own mind's reactions and inner dialogue. Be a witness, not just a doer.

5. Sharing with friends: Invite like minded persons to join you in *satsang*, or "sharing of truth," remembering that the spirit has no form, and that what is truly important is to be, more and more, Who you truly are. *Satsang* may express itself in the form of sharing of the best of what one has appreciated or realized, song, chanting, fellowship, meditation, a session of Yoga postures, a meal, any expression or gesture of love and affection.

6. Practice y*oga nidra* to gradually replace sleep with Yogic rest. Start with the practice of conscious rest when you are not fatigued, and so reduce the risk of falling asleep. Learn to allow the body to rest, while keeping your awareness in the state of Self-awareness, not withdrawn from the physical plane.

By cultivating Self-awareness in the midst of the above activities, you will experience unconditional joy, or bliss. Bliss, or *ananda* does not depend upon whether the outer circumstances are agreeable or not, whether you get what you want or what you don't want. It depends only upon your being present, in a state of awareness of how it all is.

If you can do cultivate awareness at home, you can begin to cultivate it everywhere. By practicing equanimity constantly during the highs and lows of life, the painful and pleasurable moments, the happy and unhappy times, you will gradually become a Yogi, rather than simply a consumer of spiritual materialism. You will remain in a state of Self-realization. While the spiritual market place may lose you, the world will benefit immeasurably from your enlightenment. We need more ashrams! An ashram is by definition the residence of a Yogi. So be a Yogi, and automatically your home will be an ashram!

12. Satsang

After receiving initiation into Babaji's Kriya Yoga, many persons wonder what they should do or learn next. "Practice" is the first thing, and then, "practice, practice and practice." However, because it requires some effort to move against deep-seated habits of inertia and distraction, one may become fatigued and experience a fading of interest or enthusiasm for the path. The human mind is generally very unsteady, and it often needs stimulation, something new. One remedy is "satsang," or "sharing of truth" with fellow students of yoga. The mind may resist, with doubts like "why go to a meeting with a bunch of people just like me." The answer lies in the unique chemistry that occurs when truth seekers meet one another. Jesus the Christ described it when he said: "whenever two or three of you are gathered together in my name, there I am also."

Those of the Christian faith, accept that statement simply based upon their faith. If we analyze it, and try it, the results are as replicable as those in a scientific experiment. First of all, lets identify Jesus and his name. We often confuse Jesus the person, son of Joseph (Jesus bin Joseph) with the state of realization he attained, "Christ consciousness," the "son of God." It is not an exclusive state. Jesus said: "Be ye sons of God" and "Be ye perfect, even as your Father in Heaven is perfect." Also, "all these miracles I have performed, ye shall perform even greater ones." So, when he encouraged others to gather in his name, he was referring to the Christ consciousness, the awareness that we are already enlightened, but that we need only remind ourselves of it. This is the true purpose of "satsang" as it is conceived in India.

Satsang manifests whenever we sit in the physical presence of a saint, but it can also manifest when several of us focus on our own highest truth.

How we focus on this truth, which is beyond definition and words, may vary: it may include meditation, chanting, inspirational readings, question and answer, devotional practices. The letting go of our worldly distractions for a time, allows our true self to shine forth brilliantly like the sun ("the son"). Inspiration, joy and peace flow. We recognize the divinity in ourselves and others. It is not an intellectual experience, but what our hearts longs for, the eternal moment, the infinite presence.

When, for example we really let ourselves go while chanting the names of God, what happens? Our trivial round of ego-centric preoccupations melts away into the timeless Now. When, during satsang meeting's question and answer period, we center ourselves, unprepared, and open to a higher inspiration, the ego gets out of the way and inspiration flows. We are empowered and Truth speaks through what Aurobindo referred to as the "psychic," the consciousness, which forms a bridge between our minds and God.

When we focus on words of truth, as expressed in scriptures, sacred books or inspirational literature, we also transcend the habitual perspective of a lower sense-oriented, desire oriented mind. We become attuned to that higher Consciousness which spoke through the authors of such texts.

Here is an outline for a satsang gathering:

1. Opening prayer of invocation such as "Om Kriya Babaji Nama Aum"

2. Brief introduction of everyone present;

3. Reading of some inspiration literature or sacred text;

4. Chanting of devotional chants, alternating with devotional songs individually sung;

5. Chanting of "Om Kriya Babaji Nama Aum" at least 16 times per leader, with the leadership rotating around the circle.

6. Group practice of Kriya Kundalini pranayama and meditation

7. Question and answer period;

8. Shanti mantra sung as a group

9. Sharing of a meal informally.

Feel free to add to or subtract these elements, according to the time available and your needs or interests. For example, include practice of some or all of the 18 postures. Organize satsangs on weekend outings or camping trips in natural surroundings. Organize special satsangs during holiday seasons.

May every reader pick up the telephone and call some fellow travellers of this great path of Babaji's Kriya Yoga and invite them to your home for "satsang." If you are fortunate to live in an area where such meetings are held regularly, call their organizer; if you don't know who they are consult our website directory of contact persons (www.babajiskriyayoga.net) or call or write the ashram for a reference. If you would like to attend an international satsang, attend the annual ones in Quebec, Germany, France or Brazil.

Even if you do not feel the need for fellowship with other students, I recommend you participate in it ...and regularly. The path has its ups and downs. Sometimes we don't even realize how far down we may have drifted until we participate in satsang. There will also be times when your presence will inspire others who are struggling. True spirituality is expansive in nature, and through the power of love includes others. Let your love and light shine in satsang.

13. Sacred Space

Someone recently asked me to describe my vision of the ashram (here in Quebec). The answer to this question follows. What is an ashram? It is a residence of yogis. It is not a school, nor an institute, not even a temple, for a yogi finds God everywhere and needs no special building to worship God.

For many years I have thought of creating a community of like-minded souls. I thought that this must eventually take the form of a residential community, where Kriya Yoga students would live together. That may still come about one day. We are making the facilities for that. But Master seems to have arranged for our Kriya Yoga community to manifest instead in many countries around the world, linked together spiritually, intellectually, mentally and emotionally, (and by "internet") if not always physically.

The Quebec ashram has functioned very well since 1992 as a retreat center, where thousands of people have come for initiations and retreats. It has also functioned as an ashram where many residents have come to practice Kriya Yoga and do karma yoga for long periods. It will continue to do so. To maintain it as a sacred place where anyone can become attuned to his or her greater Self has been a priority for me. It is now invested with the spiritual vibrations of so much yogic practices and experiences. In such a sacred space it is relatively easy for anyone to feel peaceful, blissful, even the presence of God.

Having been involved in the founding and maintenance of 23 yoga centers and ashrams with Yogi Ramaiah before 1989, I know how difficult it is to maintain such places. After all, we are in a physical world which is full of ignorance of the Divine Presence. People come and they go. They go when their expectations are not met, when their ego becomes threatened, when they realize how much work is required of them or when their priorities change.

I believe that investing in satsang with others is more important than investing in the bricks and mortars to build ashrams. My vision of the ashram and our community of Kriya Yoga students is that gradually a network of you will blossom into God realized yogis and that your own residences will become, therefore, by definition, ashrams.

An ashram begins with a sacred space, so do set aside at least one room if not your entire residence as sacred space, dedicated to the practice of Kriya Yoga. Avoid introducing activities there which are done without loving awareness of the Presence. Keep your space simple, functional and aesthetic. Put up pictures and wall covers which will inspire you and others. Remove anything that is unnecessary clutter. Keep the space neat and clean, ready for Babaji to visit. Light incense, oil lamps and candles. Chant the name of God as much as possible. Set aside the early mornings and evenings for sadhana, alone or with others. Regularly set aside a full 24 hours for silence, fasting and sadhana. Periodically invite others into your sacred space to practice Kriya Yoga. Read uplifting books, avoid those which only serve to distract.

Dear Readers, may you all become yogis! May sacred space overwhelm the entire world in the new Millennium! You have everything in your hands to accomplish this. You need only apply yourself to the sadhana, and your residence will become a sacred space, full of magnetic, healing, spiritual vibrations. Then all you need do to find a sacred space is to return to your own home.

PART 3

Making our life our Yoga

1. Moving towards Equilibrium: Calmly Active, Actively Calm

Our lives are often disturbed by unpredictable events. Our minds are also often invaded by thoughts, desires and fears that can be even more disturbing. These set in motion a chain reaction, which involves our emotions, speech, physiological reactions and more disturbing thoughts. It is easy to feel helpless in the face of such disturbances and later, when the storm of emotions and thoughts has subsided, feel remorse or guilt about how weak we seem to be.

What is going on? How can Yoga help us to master our human nature, so that we are not carried away by disturbing reactions?

Patanjali addresses this problem early in his Yoga-Sutras, in verse 1.16: "That freedom from the constituent forces (of nature) (which arises) due to an individual's (Self)-realization is supreme." The constituent forces of nature, the *gunas,* as they are known in the *Samkhya* philosophy underlying Yoga, are *rajas* (the tendency towards activity), *tamas* (the tendency towards inertia) and *sattva* (the tendency towards balance). Most of the time, we are moved by *rajas* or *tamas*. For example, when we feel restless, or a need to go and attend to something, it is the universal force of *rajas,* which is acting upon us. When we feel fatigue or our mind is daydreaming or confused, we are subject to that universal force of *tamas.* However, because we are ego-centered, we consider our restlessness or fatigue merely to be a personal condition and attempt to counter their influence by such things as smoking, talking, athletics, eating or drinking. While these may provide some short term compensatory effect, they do nothing to really free us from these universal forces.

Sages like Patanjali recognized this universal human dilemma, and developed the techniques of Yoga as a means of strengthening the third universal force: *sattva*. One can feel this force whenever one is calm, peaceful, content, inspired. With it comes a sense of brightness. One experiences being "calmly active, and actively calm." The practice of asana, pranayama, dhyana, mantras and bhakti increase *sattva*, and reduce the influence of *tamas* and *rajas*. Consequently, the mental fluctuations, or *vrittis*, begin to calm down, and one begins to detach from the objects of desire, which were former sources of pleasure and pain. While still subject to their memory, fantasy will arise. *Samskaras* or habitual tendencies will cause one to respond to the forces of *tamas* and *rajas*, just as in the past. So, detachment will require effort.

There is a debate between proponents of Classical Yoga, who like Patanjali recognized the need for effort to overcome the influence of the *gunas* and ones' *samskaras*, and *Advaita Vedantins*, who assert that because only the Self is real, one does not need to "do" anything to realize it, only "be." *Advaita Vedanta*, the philosophy of "non-dualism" asserts that "*tat tvam asi*," "I am That," and that the world is illusionary; therefore the practice of Yoga is not only unnecessary, but even a distraction. The Vedantin would say: because the *gunas* are only apparent, one need do nothing to counter their influence, simply be your Self. Classical Yoga grew out of the philosophies of *Vedanta* and *Samkhya*, as a practical approach to Self-realization and transformation.

Which philosophy is right? I believe it depends upon your perspective. When one is calm, centered, very present and aware, one does not need to do anything, or make any effort to realize the Self; *sattva* dominates. One need only be. But usually that is not the condition we are in. When we are stressed, agitated, restless, full of doubt, anxiety or fatigue, we need to make some effort to counter the effects of *tamas* and *rajas*, until we become permanently anchored in the state of Self-realization. Then, as Patanjali says in verse I.16, one's freedom from the *gunas* becomes supreme. When one permanently realizes the Self, the joy and peace is so fulfilling that automatically he or she gains discrimination between the Self and the non-Self, and with this loses desire for involvement even in subconscious fantasies. Desires are no longer able to have an effect. For the realized soul, detachment and desirelessness are not based on control but due to the spontaneous and constant awareness of the greater Self, all pervasive and ever joyful, in all circumstances. For the realized soul, supreme detachment is effortless.

In this state of equanimity, one no longer identifies with various desires. How to maintain it? By cultivating detachment, contentment, endurance, fearlessness, cheerfulness and adaptability in all situations. If you cannot feel this in any particular situation ask yourself "Why?" Only by truthfully answering this question will you gain permanent and effortless release from what keeps you from Self-realization.

2. What the World Needs Now is Love and Compassion

A Suffering World

The events of this past year, the war in Iraq, the genocide in the Sudan, the murder of innocents by terrorists all over the world, the incidents of American maltreatment of prisoners in Iraq and Guantanamo Bay, hurricanes, earthquakes, the latest tsunamis, have not only caused endless suffering to others, but have affected each of us all on a very deep level. The *siddha* Swami Ramalinga informs us of the great truth, which we must understand, that all souls are alike, they are all equal and related to one another. When one sees, hears, knows that one of his brothers is suffering; he too suffers, for there is a bodily relationship existing between the two. We have all experienced the Truth of this.

The problem of problems all over the world is how can we all just live a peaceful happy life? The question which arises every year is "how can we, as the people of many different nations, of different religions, languages, and cultures live together in peace and harmony?" Statesmen today debate whether the "clash of civilizations" or "clash of cultures" will inevitably bring wars. Is there an answer that can be given to every individual and to every nation tackling this problem? Perhaps, God alone knows.

The Siddhas would say that it is essential that we as individuals develop our virtue, character and our usual human faculties in order to live harmoniously and harmlessly with all in the world. Babaji tells us we can make a start by developing our character and rooting it in universal love and compassion. He gives us a framework, "focus on building character first, then on building devotion and then on obtaining Divine knowledge, then alternate your *sadhana* in service, *bhakti* and *jñana and* self-study until they interpenetrate. For there is a stage we are all capable of reaching, where Supreme Divine Love is experienced and character, devotion, and action are all perfectly aligned with Divine Will and what is expressed is always a reflection of Love and Compassion."

The Purifying Power of Love

What is this love and how can we become its instruments? Babaji tells us that Love is more than being attracted to or feeling pleasure in being with, or desiring, or even being ready to sacrifice for someone or something. Love is the source of all virtues and the source of aspiration for union. It is limitless, mysterious and miraculous. It is strength, courage and an elixir of renewal and regeneration. It is humility, patience, acceptance and endurance. It carries with it the power of expansion and transformation. We all know love in some form, so what we must do is to purify the outer expression of that love, and remove its attachment and emotion, in order to realize a true love, which permeates everything and every moment of life. There is power in the virtue of Love...power that can raise our perspective, enabling us to see the spiritual Presence within the mundane.

Sri Aurobindo says that one ray of divine love can alter the character of one's life. This love can only arise once we realize the spiritual relationship between souls, and this "love" awakens a divine energy or *shakti*, which then informs our actions with wisdom. Love is inherent in Consciousness and it manifests as we go through the process of spiritual purification, as when we let go of ignorance, egoism, attachments, and aversions. Love broadens as we embrace truth and wisdom, while engaged in activities of the world. It is not so difficult to love God as He who rules over all and is above everything earthly. What is difficult and necessary is to love the Lord manifested in every form, in every man.

Babaji tells us that compassion is a natural expression of the inner state of the soul, when the soul is at peace. Our pure inner state is a dynamic force and its vibration of peace can benefit the world at large. Compassion, like love, is a quality of the heart and a virtue of the soul. It develops as our hearts open to our connection with the Lord and with others. So, how can the deeply religious hate? The Siddhas tell us that it takes a constant awareness of oneself, a constant *sadhana* of self-reflection and detachment along with the development of the virtues of love and compassion to progressively rid oneself of all hatred. So, how can the deeply religious not be always compassionate? Normally man is so concerned with his own sense of lack that he feels he cannot afford to be compassionate with others. Only a strong spiritual discipline can create the mental order necessary to develop the equanimity and compassion, which expands love to include others, rather than to exclude them. The Mother of Sri Aurobindo Ashram said, "compassion seeks to relieve the suffering of all, whether they deserve it or not."

By identifying with others and enlarging one's world to embrace all others, true compassion is cultivated. Only by cultivating dispassion can one truly embrace everyone. For only a truly dispassionate mind can be peaceful and free from the fear, sorrow, worry, hatred and guilt to which mankind is subjected. With a dispassionate mind one can be courageous enough to live lovingly and compassionately with all others. Freedom, love and compassion expand and one begins to embrace the interests of others. One begins to understand their perspective, and ultimately identifies with them as brother and sister and serves them, as one is able.

How can dispassion purify?

By practicing dispassion, compassion will arise in stages. First in your thoughts, then with all those you come in contact with in your daily life, and then with all those in your communities, and finally with all those in the world. An outpouring of love from your heart will grow and grow and you will become open to the immense power underlying Compassion, which can transform everything. For compassion is a force of God, a virtue of God, not a virtue of any religion.

How do I develop dispassion?

Reject even the slightest anxiety, sorrow, anger, jealousy; any disturbance of the mind. Do not allow for any excuse or justification for a disturbing thought, no matter how plausible or justifiable it might seem to be. Remember that in any mental disturbance, it is always the prana that is disturbed. Try to separate yourself from the troubled prana and keep yourself centered in your highest nature. Reject the hold that fear, desire, aversion or attachment may have on you. Reject even an emotion coming from your "heart," if it is causing the disturbance.

Sri Aurobindo says, "If the source of a mental disturbance is your will or intelligence then it will be harder to control the disturbance." Consciously align your will and intelligence towards the goal of dispassion.

While all of our yogic sadhana including *asana, bandhas, pranayama, mantra, and meditation* involves purification and will develop dispassion to some extent, true dispassion requires us to go beyond the egoistic sense of "I and mine." Dispassion really asks us to get beyond the sense of being the doer. Only in this way can we remain centered in calm heart-filled awareness, regardless of the circumstances we find our self.

3. Judgment, or How to Avoid Harming Others and Ourselves

In the 1970's there was a best seller, entitled "I'm O.K., you're O.K." which like many books since then, dealt with human relationships, and how to make the most of them. The title expresses what most of us do unconsciously all the time: make judgments about others. Unfortunately, most of our judgments are not "O.K." but rather, they express opinions, which harm others and ourselves. Consequently, our human relationships become a source of great division and conflict. In past decades much of psychology has focused upon improving our social relations, managing conflict, and making our personalities more acceptable socially. The role of judgments in our social relations, however, is not widely understood.

Empathy and antipathy

Studies in psychology have revealed that most persons form fairly accurate impressions of others within a few moments. It is as if the human being is able to quickly scan others and absorb, even intuitively, many valid factors. However, these impressions provoke reactions that are usually colored by one's own tendencies and feelings, which in turn create judgments. For example, a recent study of people being interviewed revealed that interviewees who felt empathy for their interviewers, tended to be selected for the position, even though their answers and qualifications were often not adequate, while interviewees who felt some dislike or antipathy for the interviewer did not succeed, even when their answers and qualification were exceptionally good. This indicates that the interviewers formed judgments about the interviewees based upon subjective factors, including emotions, even intuition, more than upon objective facts. In other words, we have the ability to sense the judgments others have about us.

Judgment defined

Judgments are opinions that develop on the basis of limited experiences, even hearsay. Someone shares some gossip about someone else, and we jump to a conclusion, we judge. The problem with judgments is that they are not based upon facts and they tend to solidify before available facts are assessed. Even worse, too often they are based upon prejudice, fear and imagination. For example, do you have an immediate response to seeing young Muslim men in a crowded airport or subway train? Or do you react upon seeing two men, or a man and woman who are of different races speaking intimately?

Judgments are in short incomplete opinions, based upon too little information, usually first impressions, imagination and past associations. They reflect our prejudices and preferences. We tend to see what we want to see or what we fear. As such, judgments are motivated by subconscious factors, which drive us unconsciously.

Good judgment

Our challenge is not so much to avoid making judgments, but rather learning how to develop "good judgment." "Good judgment" is a much admired quality, and its origins are not well understood. It is the product of reflection, and is imbued with common sense, if not wisdom. It is notably free of emotion and prejudice. It is also perspicacious, in that it attempts to weigh all relevant factors. It is "good" because it is edifying to all concerned. It uplifts, brings joy. It never harms. A friend may say something truthful to another friend, which the other is not ready to hear. Then, it is rejected, and there is conflict, even loss of friendship. So "good judgment" expresses itself in a way that seeks to free all concerned of suffering, if not to find joy. It is the product of a mind, which has access to the truth of a situation either through intuition, experience, or strong analytical skills. Good judgment is the result most often of experience, and so elders are usually considered to be imbued with it, more than young persons, whose judgments are too often imbued with emotional excitement or rebelliousness. Moreover, "good judgment" is attributed to the wise, who seem to have a special connection to the truth of things, an intuitive ability to touch the ground of being, that which outlives everything else.

Why are judgments harmful?

Judgments are generally harmful for three reasons. First, they reflect the state of mind of the person forming it. Psychological studies have revealed that more than two thirds of the time, the average person is in a negative mental or emotional state. Feelings of depression, grief, anger, fear, impatience, and pride rule the average person. Until or unless one has learned to master these states, judgment is usually an expression of one's own state. That is, we project onto others, what we ourselves are experiencing. We assume that they are experiencing what we are experiencing because our perceptions are colored by our own internal state. They harm the other by projecting onto them a negative, if not erroneous reaction.

Secondly, judgments are harmful because they assume a static condition. When we express a judgment about another person, there is an implicit assumption that the person judged is unlikely to change. While human nature is generally habitual, it is often erratic. People have bad days, tragedies, and emotional outbursts. Such behavior is atypical, and does not reflect the person's underlying character. So forming a judgment about a person who is having a difficult day or acting outside their usual character, is erroneous. Also, young people do grow up overcoming immature behavior. The strong-willed overcome bad behavioral tendencies and reform themselves. Therefore judgments do not allow for growth, for change in a positive direction, and are therefore harmful. Judgment typically confuses the person with their behavior.

Wisdom is needed to perceive the difference between the person and their behavior. With wisdom comes the realization that we are not our body, mind and personality; rather, these aspects of us, are like clothing, which can be changed, or kept out of habit. With wisdom, we realize that a person's true identity is pure consciousness, the soul, the Seer or Witness, and that it has the power to change habitual behavior by exercising it's will.

Third, and most important, judgments are harmful because they reinforce the quality condemned, not only in the person being judged, but also, and most significantly in the one who is judging. When we form a judgment about another, for example, thinking, "that person is so greedy," we are actually dwelling upon the quality of greed, and are therefore strengthening it within ourselves. Like worry, which can be defined as "meditating upon what you don't want," judgment of others is often like meditating upon what you do not like in yourself.

Patanjali, one of the fathers of Classical Yoga, and a contemporary of Jesus said: "By cultivating attitudes of friendship towards the happy, compassion towards the unhappy, delight in the virtuous, and equanimity towards the non-virtuous, the consciousness returns to its undisturbed calmness." (Yoga Sutras I.33) When we do not do this, what happens? Our minds become disturbed by judgment, ill feelings, resentment, anger, and disgust. Consequently, we lose the fundamental requirement necessary for God realization: calm, peace, inner purity and innocence. The world is within us. To change the world from a place of evil to a "kingdom of heaven" we can and must change our thoughts. We must learn to forgive the lapses of others and not dwell on their weakness.

Ahimsa, non-harming, the antidote for judgment

How to avoid making judgments which harm others? The wise tell us that we need to develop an attitude of non-harming, which in India is referred to as "ahimsa." It includes thoughts, words and actions. It is based upon the recognition that there are consequences or karma, which results even from thoughts. Thoughts, often repeated form habits, and habits then direct one's life. If the habit involves desire, and the desire is not satisfied, one becomes confused as to the source of happiness in life, that is, the ever existent inner joy of the soul.

Jesus said at his crucifixion: "Father, forgive them, for they know not what they do," speaking of those who had condemned him to such a terrible ordeal. Rather than dwelling on his own pain or asking God to condemn those who had condemned him, Jesus was more concerned with the karmic consequences of his persecutors' actions. He apparently knew, that according to the law of karma, the consequences would be severe, and he did not want them to suffer because of him. So, he asked his Father to forgive them. Forgiveness springs from love, not judgment. It was a supreme example of what Patanjali recommended, in Yoga Sutras: "When filled with negative thoughts or feelings, cultivate their opposite." It also allowed Jesus to find peace, and to free himself from the corrosive effects of anger.

Blessing and loving others are always better alternatives to judging. Our thoughts and prayers have significant effects on others, and we can really make a difference in the lives of others by our good thoughts and blessings. On an occult level, thought forms have a life of their own. When we think of others, good or ill, we produce thought forms that attach themselves to these persons and influence their behavior and experiences. After discovering that her husband had been unfaithful to her, only a few weeks after their marriage, one young woman prayed that he would die. A few days later, he died violently in a traffic accident, and his head was decapitated. The young bride was so distraught with feelings of guilt that for over a year thereafter, she pretended that he was still living with her, and prepared his meals and served him as if he was, until her family convinced her to seek psychological counselling.

Researchers at Duke University, in the USA, have been able to verify that prayer is effective in helping the sick to recover from illness, often miraculously. In most cases, the time required for convalescence is greatly reduced when others pray for our recovery. On an occult level, prayer generates powerful thought forms that can directly help others. A woman critically hurt in a traffic accident recognized a total stranger who had prayed for her at the crash scene when the stranger came to check on her in the hospital. The woman claimed that it was this stranger's prayers, which had brought her back. So, we should, as matter of routine, bless others, pray for others, silently and anonymously whenever we see anyone suffering in some way. We all have many occasions to do so. Even in traffic, when someone cuts us off or has car trouble, or when a passer-by appears sad or troubled, we can say "May God bless this person." Or "May God help this person to find peace," or "to slow down," or "to find happiness." We can rejoice with others in their good fortune, rather than feeling jealous: "God has blessed this person. May they continue to be blessed, and share their blessings with others."

Final Judgment or Forgiveness? Sayings and parables from Jesus

Jesus said: "With the measure that you judge others, so shall you be judged." (Matthew 7:1-2) Jesus was challenging the religious norm of that time. Judaism was a legalistic religion. God was the Lawgiver, and he gave the Ten Commandments to Moses, on Mt. Sinai. God was the ultimate judge, and He was believed to condemn those who transgressed his laws, and to reward those who respected them. This was an advance over other religions such as that of the Canaanites, who worshipped an idol in the form of a golden calf. Primitive religions are motivated by fear. Especially fear of death or pain. So, primitive man tries to appease with sacrifices, what he regards as supernatural sources for natural events and phenomena, and which threaten his life. Later, when people organize themselves into societies, to avoid harming one another, societies develop laws to govern human behavior with social norms. Because such laws need an ultimate authority, the rulers, generally kings or chiefs, attribute their authority to God. Also, to preserve a sense of justice, man creates an image of God who is just, and who is the ultimate judge, punishing the wicked and rewarding the righteous. For example, we find in the Old Testament, many of the prophets speaking of the "Final Judgment," and in India, the concept of *"prarabha karma,"* wherein the actions of ones life bringing consequences into the next one. So, people from this stage of religion, attempt to balance their sins, or bad karma, with things that will atone for their transgressions. The means for doing so may be as simple as penance, voluntary self-denial, or in medieval Christianity, with indulgences, contributions to the Church, which would allow their sins to be forgiven.

Jesus said: "Why do you notice the sliver in your friend's eye, but overlook the log in your own? How can you say to your friend, 'Let me get the sliver out of your eye,' when there is that log in your own? You phoney, first take the log out of your own eye and then you'll see well enough to remove the sliver from your friend's eye." (Matthew 7: 3-5) In other words, critics should concentrate on correcting themselves. Furthermore, he said: "Don't imagine that I have come not to end the Law or the Prophets, but to fulfil them." (Matthew 5:17-20) What does this mean? Jesus was not saying ignore the law, but realize that God loves you. Repeatedly, Jesus tells us parables, like that of the prodigal son, (in Luke 15:11-32) to illustrate this "gospel" or "good news." Because God loves you, you can love others. And a God who loves you cannot condemn you to eternal damnation! This was his most important teaching. He repeatedly exhorted his disciples and audiences to love one another, to purify themselves of material attachments, in order to enter the kingdom of heaven, which he said was all around us, if only we could develop the purity of vision to see it. (Luke 17:20-21, Matthew 18:2). We must become as innocent as little children, Jesus said, if we want to enter this ever present kingdom of heaven. He said: "Love your enemies, and pray for those who persecute you." (Luke 6.27) He said: "If someone strikes you on one cheek, offer to them the other as well to strike." (Luke 6.29) So love supersedes the law and judgment. You may have the right to claim "an eye for an eye" as the Old Testament prophets claimed, but as Mahatma Gandhi, said: "An eye for an eye ultimately leaves the whole world blind." That is, when we are blinded by judgment and retribution, we fail to see that ultimately, we are all members of one human family, and that through love, all differences can be overcome.

Mahatma Gandhi: modern apostle of non-violence

Mahatma Gandhi said: "All sins are committed in secrecy. The moment we realize that God witnesses even our thoughts we shall be free." That is, sin is the absence of awareness of the presence of God. Therefore, judging others for their sins, blinds us to our own! Gandhi was a self-professed student of truth, who, after forty years of struggle, in 1947 finally forced the British Empire to quit India without violence, by bringing the ancient principle of "ahimsa" or "non-harming." He developed his methods by studying Jainism, and the parables of Jesus, which puts emphasis on non-harming. Jain monks, wear a mask over their mouths, and sweep the ground before them, to avoid inadvertently killing even insects. His methods of non-harming, or ahimsa became the basis of the civil rights movement used by Martin Luther King in the USA in the 1960's and other labor and social movements, which used passive resistance and non-violent protests and demonstrations to sensitize the public to their causes. In India, thousands of men and women pledged themselves to his satyagraha movement, wherein they dedicated themselves to living according to principles of truth (satya) without harming others. In large demonstrations against the British colonial army, thousands of them were clubbed to death or maimed without the least resistance. So staunch were they in "turning the other cheek," that the British at last were forced to give up over 300 years of colonial rule in India. Gandhi spent decades in British prisons, fasting for long periods, to demonstrate his resistance to the British and their policies. When he campaigned against the importation of British textiles to India, he won the sympathy of even the British textile workers, whose own jobs had been lost because of India's boycott. His life and methods, demonstrated that we do not have to judge others to beat them! We need only take a firm stand in our convictions, and seek mutual accommodation without harming others, to gain their sympathy and understanding. He said: "The hardest heart and the grossest ignorance must disappear before the rising sun of suffering without anger and without malice."

Gandhi said: "Non-violence is the law of our species as violence is the law of the brute. The spirit lies dormant in the brute and he knows no law but that of physical might. The dignity of man requires obedience to a higher law - to the strength of the spirit." And: "It is a force that may be used by individuals as well as by communities. It may be used as well in political as in domestic affairs. Its universal applicability is a demonstration of its permanence and invincibility. It can be used alike by men, women and children. It is totally untrue to say that it is a force to be used only by the weak so long as they are not capable of meeting violence by violence."

In speaking of the political movement which he founded to free India, he said "Satyagraha is gentle, it never wounds. It must not be the result of anger or malice. It is never fussy, never impatient, never vociferous. It is the direct opposite of compulsion. It was conceived as a complete substitute for violence."

Seeing unity in the diversity

So, judgment, whether it pertains to our personal feelings about others, or how we view God and our soul's ultimate trajectory, does not have the final word. The wise, the compassionate, the spiritual heroes of our civilization, from Buddha to Jesus, to Mahatma Gandhi, have discovered that love, forgiveness, compassion and non-harming, supersede it. So, if judgment costs you your peace of mind, it costs too much. If it harms others, it reverberates within you too. The Yoga masters, the wise Siddhas, called God "goodness," and declared that we are all part of one family, one land. The wise, see what is good in others, and turn away from the rest. Judgment divides. Love unites. Love and forgiveness overtake the law, and bring about a new perspective, in which we see the essential unity of all.

4. Yoga as a Social Movement

For more than 100 years Indian Yogis have been teaching in the West. Their influence has been profound, despite the fact that there has been little acknowledgement of this by historians, sociologists, politicians or the media. Where the influence has been noticed, for example, by the leaders of Western religious institutions, it has been usually in the form of alarm. Western religious institutions have felt threatened by the teachings of Yoga, fearing that they will lose influence, or out of ignorance, that there is something harmful or un-Christian about an Eastern spiritual practice.

This is really nothing new. Organized religions have always sought to maintain their power base and to increase their influence at the expense of their members. It is in the nature of any institution to put its own needs and position ahead of the needs of its members, for which it was organized originally. Organized religious institutions are generally fear and guilt based enterprises, which maintain their power by first warning of the danger of hell, the devil, or damnation, and then offer an insurance policy against such imagined threats, usually a set of beliefs or rituals, which are supposed to nullify the effects of one's bad behavior, termed "sin" in Western circles, or "karma," in eastern circles.

Those who follow seriously a spiritual path, however, find themselves on a mostly solitary route. While mystics may have fellow travellers or guides along the way, this usually occurs only for relatively short periods. Historically, when they joined together to form monasteries or communities, they may, for a while have been tolerated by the prevailing religious institutions around them, but they were never fully trusted. This can be seen, for example, in the case of the empty monasteries all over Italy today. Four hundred years ago, they were filled and vibrant with mystics. But a mystic does not need a priest, much less a pope, because he/she can communicate directly with the Lord, through the contemplative methods of their order. So, while tolerated for a time, such communities were not encouraged by the Church. Monasteries have gradually emptied, as people began to put more faith in science and technology, and less and less in religion.

A mystic, which is the Christian term for Yogi, is not unaware of society's ills. Nor would a mystic ignore society. Because of one's expanded consciousness, and the wide-opening of their heart chakra, a mystic is even more sensitive than most. But how can a mystic express himself/herself in contemporary society? Mystics are often looked upon with much suspicion, and because of their practices and experiences, even with fear, born of ignorance.

How then can the modern mystic, as solitary as he or she is, expect to have any influence on society? Must they organize to do so? Is Yoga an actual social movement, or only potentially so?

"No man is an island" said John Donne, the English poet, and this applies to the mystic or Yogi. In Classical Yoga, the first limb, the "yamas" or restraints, govern the Yogis social behavior: non-harming, non-stealing, non-lying, greedlessness and chastity. These are observed not to satisfy some moral principles, but because their observance is both a prerequisite for, and an expression of the enlightened state. By observing them one comes to experience that there is no "other," but only One. The ultimate social state.

The determined observance of these restraints by a number of dedicated Yogis can and will have a profound impact upon society. And this does not even require that one become a political leader, as in the case of Mahatma Gandhi, who was a Kriya Yogi, and the father of the non-violence movement, which gave birth to India's independence, the American Civil Rights movement, and the ending of apartheid in South Africa. In any social interchange, whether it is with family members, work colleagues, clients, supervisors, or strangers, there is an interchange of energy. That energy may be infused with love and compassion, which is profoundly yogic by definition, or infused with anger, greed, impatience, competition or antipathy. We may feed one another with our love and compassion, helping one another to be who we truly are, conscious, universal beings, or we may poison one another with our egoistic tendencies. On the contrary, the determined observance of their opposite, for example, by the extremists in the Israeli-Palestinian conflict, and in Northern Ireland, the Catholic-Protestant conflict, produces only unending sorrow. One can imagine that if the Palestinians had also adopted a non-violent approach to national liberation, they would have gotten their own nation thirty years ago.

Yoga is a social movement, for it seeks to awaken and to transform one human being at a time from the ordinary egoistic state. Our modern pluralistic culture is largely inspired by the principles of individualism, materialism and consumerism, which amount to a recipe for egoism. To the extent that one practices Yoga, beginning with the restraints or *yamas* (cited above) and observances, the *niyamas* (purity, contentment, self-study, intense practice, and devotion to the Lord) one is engaged in a kind of guerrilla war against the prevailing culture. The word "culture" is derived from the Latin word "culte" which means "worship." So, in our modern materialistic, consumer, individualistic culture, most members of society worship or value, above all, those things that are material, which can be consumed and which enhance their feeling of being special.

A Yogi on the other hand values or worships the Lord, the Absolute Reality, and this is found within, in the spiritual plane of existence, initially, until, in the enlightened state, one begins to perceive it in everything transcendentally. He does not feel that he is anything special, and does not even see himself as the "doer." The Yogi recognizes the hand of the Lord guiding and empowering at every stage.

How to change this perspective is the concern of Yoga, and while it is the responsibility of each practitioner to raise himself up (by his own efforts), there is an undeniable aid which is provided between members of the Yoga community or *sangha*. The word *sangha*, or in Tamil, *sangam*, means literally, the place where rivers meet. So, each of us is a river, in this sense, and when we meet there is an exchange. When a person is discouraged or confused, and this may occur even in the case of Yoga adepts with much experience, the presence of fellow Yogis, will usually serve to heal or inspire. While this exchange is most clearly seen in the exchange of vital energy between two people, a kind word or thought on the mental plane, a bit of advice on the intellectual plane, or a smile and expression of joy on the spiritual plane may be enough to remove the discouragement or confusion. It is therefore essential that all practitioners of Yoga, not isolate themselves as a rule. By sharing their love and compassion they learn to integrate their spiritual realizations at all levels of existence, to overcome egoism, and to serve as a pure instrument for the Divine, in bringing about a more compassionate, conscious and divinely inspired society.

While as many as 20 million people in North America, by some estimates are now practicing Yoga, and ninety percent of these practice it only as a physical exercise, this does not mean that the influence of Yoga is limited only to the fields of health or physical fitness. If one continues to practice Yoga, the effects begin to include the nervous system and the mind, and consequently there is an expansion of consciousness into the spiritual dimension. This occurs even without trying, as a natural and spontaneous effect. What begins as a physical need, or a means to control the effects of stress, eventually becomes a very personal spiritual path. A spiritual path leads one to increasing levels of personal freedom from the round of habitual tendencies fostered by our social conditioning. As we begin the constant practice of detachment (*vairagya*) we begin to let go of what we are not, including our social conditioning, and experience who we truly are. The experience of Self-realization replaces the confusion of egoism, the habit of identifying with what we are not: thoughts, emotions, memories, habits, and sensations. As our consciousness expands we become a witness, and perhaps the Witness. "I am a man, a professional, black, white or asian" says the ego. "I am That I am" says the awakened Yogi. The social implications of such a change in consciousness are profound and wide-ranging. Not only does the Yogi become a source of peace and well-being for those who enjoy his or her company, but a dynamo of energy, guided by unusual clarity and insight. Such a person can and will act as a powerful agent for the Good, solving the problems of this world in a spirit of compassion and wisdom.

We live in a period of history wherein the interdependence of everyone on the planet has never been so great. This social crisis, wherein a flu epidemic or an act of suicide in one part of the world, can instantly affect the economy and political stability of society on the other side of the planet, requires nothing less than the discipline of Yoga by millions of inspired practitioners. The media has become the greatest tool of those who would seek to terrorize society. A great defence against terrorism is Yoga, for it strikes down at its source, the fear, which permits terrorism to be effective. Fear is simply imagination of the possibility of suffering, without evaluating the probability of its occurrence. This requires mental discipline, the practice of detachment, and the calm clear thinking, which Yoga inspires. Furthermore, the societal effect of a powerful yogi's positive thinking or blessing, is more powerful than the dispersed negative thinking of a thousand ordinary folk.

May Yoga practitioners all come to recognize the power that they have to bring peace and enlightened solutions to the diverse problems in the world.

5. "All countries are my homeland and all persons are part of my family"

In 1997, after returning from three months of foreign travel in six countries, in which more than a 14 initiation seminars were conducted I could really feel in my heart the above famous saying of the Eighteen

Tamil Yoga Siddhas. However, one does not need to travel as much as I do to get a sense of how closely connected everyone on the planet now is. Just move into cyberspace and you are in touch with millions of persons around the world.

The great French philosopher, André Malraux opined during the Cold War that "the next century will be spiritual or it will not be at all." One does not need to look very far for evidence of what doomsayers are predicting before the beginning of the next millenium. And seers including Nostradamus, Edgar Cayce and even Yogananda have predicted terrible catastrophes during the next years. There are a growing number of indicators that such predictions are coming true: the effects of global warming, earthquakes, massive forest fires, genocidal wars, epidemics of bird flu, HIV and other new diseases, international terrorists and religious fanatics with weapons of mass destruction poised to wipe out millions.

I am frequently asked what do I think of such prophecies and what should one do? On the eve of this new millennium, what many predict will be a period of great destruction, I wish to reassure you of my firm conviction that if all of us continue to practice Babaji's Kriya Yoga. for the benefit of everyone on this planet, as the Tamil Siddhas did, whatever catastrophes or destruction bound to occur in the coming years will be greatly mitigated. We will serve as part of the solution to bring about a new era of world peace and harmony.

This is not to say that we can continue to conduct our lives as we have in the past. Rather it is a wake-up call to re-dedicate ourselves to our yogic practices and reach out to others all around us. This must also include the remembrance of the Divine in all of our relationships, and setting aside more time to go deep within, into our silent source from which all our strength and inspiration may be found.

With this perspective, at the end of 1994, I left my 25 year career to dedicate myself fulltime to making Babaji's Kriya Yoga available to persons all over the world. Through Babaji's grace I have trained teachers of Kriya Yoga in nearly ten countries and developed an ongoing mission in a dozen others, with nearly 15,000 students initiated to date.

I would like to share with the reader my first "pilgrimage to Russia", October 20-24, 1997. It was very moving for me, nearly as moving as my first visit to India in 1972. Even though I have been a life long student of foreign affairs, nothing that I had read about Russia prepared me for what I experienced there in October. I went with much apprehension as to the physical conditions there, the readiness of potential students and about how I would manage to communicate the beauty of Babaji's Kriya Yoga.

Upon arrival, I could not help but think of my last visit to Eastern Europe, in 1968, when I had been arrested in East Berlin, imprisoned and interrogated for many hours in the former Gestapo headquarters for inadvertently getting to close to the "Wall," which divided the eastern and western halves of the city. And despite the fact that the arrangements for my visit had all easily been arranged via internet with Sergei, the trip was nearly cancelled at the last minute because of bureaucratic delays in obtaining a visa. Nearly 30 years later, arriving in Moscow's dark and forbidding international airport, and walking into the crowd outside the exit gate my apprehensions began to melt away when I was greeted by three smiling faces, who introduced themselves as Sergei, Ira, and Galya.

Later, as we left the airport in Galya's old Lada, I got a taste of Russian humor: "We expected you to be dressed all in white. We followed another passenger who was, until we realized that we had the wrong person."

We drove directly to an elementary school through streets which had surprisingly few cars, where I was scheduled to give an introductory lecture. Inside the classroom there were 28 Russians waiting expectantly, sitting in a circle. Some of them had made a small altar and lit some candles. I placed Babaji's picture on it and we began to chant "Om Kriya Babaji Nama Aum." It was thrilling for me to feel His presence in this place. Then I gave a lecture on Babaji and his Kriya Yoga, speaking slowly so that the translator Sergei Gavrilov could keep up. Later I learned that they had come from all over the former Soviet Union: from Kazakstan, the Urals, Belorussia, even the pacific coast of Siberia. Most of them had already read the Russian translation of "Babaji and the 18 Siddha Kriya Yoga Tradition," which had been published in Moscow just one year before.

The lecture struck a sympathic chord in their hearts and the group radiated a glow of love and appreciation for the message I had to deliver to them. Most of them were in their 40's, and I sensed all of them had been through a lot of hardship, particularly since the collapse of the Soviet Union and its economy during the past three years. After the lecture, we drove a few miles to Red Square and the Kremlin, walking into it in a light rain just as the clock struck midnight. I marvelled at being there amongst the huge walls and St. Basil's Cathedral, symbol of the Czar's empire. We went into a small chapel at the other end of the square where we viewed ancient icons of the Madonna and child, all framed in gold, brilliantly lit up, and pulsating with spiritual vibrations which reminded me of some temples of India.

During the three following days I visited several churches and monasteries, and travelled all over Moscow. Despite 70 years of being dominated by the Communist regime, the spiritual heritage of the Russian Orthodox Church is palpable in the lives of many Russians. I found many Russians to be deeply spiritual, full of love and wisdom. What is happening there seemed to be like "springtime," with many old things lying around lifeless, like leaves on the ground after the snow melts, and here and there, new enterprises, stores, renovations, and spiritual movements, like beautiful flowers beginning to sprout.

Returning to the apartment of my host, Ira, late each night after the seminar, I was moved to see so many old persons in the subway stations struggling to survive by peddling packages of American cigarettes, toilet paper, or household articles, their faces red and bloated by the effects of alcohol and the cold.

On the other hand, I was impressed with the determination and vision of younger persons to create a new society based upon cooperation, technology and spiritual sciences. I could appreciate their perspective: highly trained in science and engineering, and deeply spiritual, despite daunting odds, my new Russian friends are determined to make a lasting contribution to the world. I am sure with such people there, we can expect great things from Russia in the 21st Century.

The initiation seminar was given during the evenings, from 7 to 11 p.m. in a classroom of a public school. Twenty-six persons received initiation. The students were sincere and many of them did very well in their practice of breathing, meditation and postures. A Moscow group was formed and monthly meetings scheduled. Tentative plans were made for a second level initiation after one year.

Jai Babaji! Jai Kriya Yoga! May the fragrance of Tamil Kriya Yoga Siddhantham spread all over the world.

6. Holy Madness, Kundalini, Shakti pat and Ego-Crushing

I recently read Georg Feurestein's book "Holy Madness - The Shock Tactics and Radical Teachings of Crazy-Wise Adepts, Holy Fools and Rascal Gurus," which was gifted to me by the author. It is a valuable work for the modern student of Yoga who may at some point encounter the type of enigmatic teacher, which is described in this book. After recounting the stories and place of such remarkable personalities down through the ages in various spiritual traditions, the author related the stories of several modern day examples, such as Gurdjieff, Rajneesh, Chogyam Trungpa Rimpoche, Swami Nityananda and his own crazy wise guru, Adi Da (Bubba Free John). It is a remarkably balanced and perceptive analysis of the value and pitfalls of following such a teacher.

It was meaningful for me, especially since my own teacher, Yogi Ramaiah, was such a "crazy-wise" adept. He often referred to himself as "a madcap yogi," and while he generally followed a strict discipline, he was a master at creating difficult situations for his students, wherein they would be confronted with their own worst reactions: fear, resentment, pride, embarrassment, insecurity, frustration, confusion. Laughter seemed to be the best remedy, and we often said that it would be impossible to tell someone else what it had been like. His behavior was usually enigmatic. Congratulations to Georg for delivering so much understanding in between two covers.

Some notable quotes: "Accepting the fact that our appraisal of a teacher is always subjective so long as we have not ourselves attained his or her level of spiritual accomplishment, there is at least one important criterion that we can look for in a guru: does he or she genuinely promote disciples' personal and spiritual growth, or does he or she obviously or ever so subtly undermine their maturation? Would-be disciples should take a careful, level-headed look at the community of students around their prospective guru. They should especially scrutinize those who are closer to the guru than most."

"Whether teachings experienced along the way are beautiful and pleasant, or unpleasant and harsh, or even bland, all are grist for the mill of awakening. The slightest reaction reflects the subtlest clinging. It is a meaningful clue to where you are still holding on. Simply watching your reaction makes anything a teaching."

"Accountability and responsibility are important instruments of balance in the spiritual process that takes place between teacher and disciple. When they are scorned we find power games and abuse, as has been amply demonstrated in recent years by the fallen angels of spiritual and religious life in America and elsewhere."

"My personal conviction is that, in due course, our age will develop its own characteristic spirituality and that this will give rise to a new class of spiritual guide. The traditional guru type, I submit, is generally too autocratic and paternalistic for our modern sensibilities. Hence the Eastern-style guru-centric approaches are bound to fail in the West, obliging us to look at alternatives. Those who are spiritually "musical" will look and call for new maestros - teachers who are also learners, who wear their halos lightly, and who do not mind sticking their feet in the humus of life in order to walk with their fellow beings, including those who are not of the privileged white middle class."

"So despite the misgivings expressed about traditional crazy-wise adepts and eccentric masters in this book, they can conceivably still serve a useful societal function: to act as mirrors of the "insanity" of consensus reality and as beacons of that larger Reality that we habitually tend to exclude from our lives. To the extent that they can help us free ourselves from the blinders with which we block out Reality and conceal ourselves (or our Self) from ourselves, we would do well to heed their message. At the same time, I feel, they are relics of an archaic spirituality that, sooner or later, will be replaced by a more integrated approach to self-transcendence. This new approach will be sustained by teachers, including holy fools, who place personal growth and integrity above the need to instruct, Reality above traditional fidelity, and compassion and humor above all role-playing."

The above reflects the approach, which I have attempted to implement, since leaving a "crazy wisdom" teacher. I believe that our students have been the big winners to the extent they have applied themselves to the practice. While many have not appreciated what they have received, I know that only a fraction are prepared to invest the time and effort required to go far in this field.

Shaktipat or transmission by gurus

Several past and present "masters" from India have succeeded in attracting a lot of attention and followers to themselves by promising to give what is sometimes referred to as "*shaktipat*," or the transmission of energy resulting in altered states of consciousness. Swami Muktananda and Yogi Amrit Desai are two examples of those who did this for many years. Often the recipients did experience altered states of consciousness, or uncontrolled movements of their body, even hurling like a dog. Even worse, some suffered long lasting psychotic states, and permanent deranged states of consciousness. The record was not good, and the reputations of both these teachers were seriously damaged.

My teacher always used to say with respect to promises of spiritual experiences or "*shaktipat*," "to put more faith in your own sadhana than in such promises." There are many reasons for this: First, our human nature, with all of its *samskaras* or habits, resists change. Therefore, even after having a so called experience of energy or whatever, one returns to ones habitual state of consciousness and neuroses. Secondly, nowhere in the yogic literature is "*shaktipat*" recommended as a means of acquiring lasting change in consciousness. Patanjali tells us that with regards to our deep-seated subconscious desires and tendencies, the *samskaras*, that it is only by repeatedly returning to the source, that is, by returning to the samadhi state that we can uproot them. Thirdly, such a promise leaves one dependent upon the "master," whereas the objective is to make oneself a master of one's own, body, life, and mind. Fourth, it gives the impression that "enlightenment'" can be purchased for the cost of a seminar, or as a result of an experience. Whereas, enlightenment, or the establishment of one's consciousness in the state of Self-realization known as *samadhi*, is rarely attained, and only as a result of a long process of disciplined sadhana or practice of spiritual or yogic disciplines, with practically no exceptions. Fifth, any experience is in the physical, vital or mental plane, and as such, is limited in time and effect. In the spiritual plane, one goes beyond experiences, time and space, and realizes pure consciousness. This alone is the goal of Yoga and all authentic spiritual traditions. Sixth, to claim that one can transmit enlightenment to someone else as a result of shaktipat is deceptive. There are no shortcuts to "enlightenment." Finally, no truly "enlightened" teacher would make any claim of specialness, or superiority over others. When one reaches the enlightened state, there is no "other;" one has gone beyond the need to have or give any experience because there is no longer an experiencer. One is one with the Supreme truth, transcendent to all experiences and forms. One enlightened teacher, Ramana Maharshi would not even acknowledge a guru disciple relationship between himself and others.

What is important for everyone to remember is that our sadhana includes not only a transcendence or vertical ascent into the spiritual, but also horizontal integration of Self-realization into all the areas of our life.

Ego-crushing by gurus

During the past seven years of research, translation and study of the literature of the Eighteen Yoga Siddhas, I have nowhere found any encouragement for what is commonly referred to as "ego-crushing" by gurus as a method of transforming their students. One could define "ego-crushing" as any action or word by a guru, which is done with the intention of creating a reaction in a disciple that will be difficult for that disciple to manage.

For example, the guru might publicly blame the disciple for some failure, even when there is no justification. The disciple has to master the desire to become defensive, which is one of the many masks of fear. Not only is "ego-crushing" not mentioned in the works of Patanjali, Boganathar, Ramalinga and Tirumular, it is not found in the writings of any of the lesser known Eighteen Yoga Siddhas. In observing its effects on myself and my brother and sister disciples, I have observed that this method in most cases, drives disciples away, and in some, left scars so deep, they have not yet healed. Even with those who remained with my teacher until the end of his life, it is evident that as a method of eradicating, even reducing the ego, its effectiveness is very debatable.

I have come to believe that the risk that "ego-crushing" becomes abusive rather than supportive to a student's growth is too great. There can be a fine line between abuse and support, which depends not only upon the student's ability and willingness to become a disciple and in that role, to grow in each instance, but it also depends on the state of mind of the guru. If the guru has even the slightest preference, then it is coming from his or her ego. I have come to believe that the ideal support of a teacher is his/her presence and consciousness in the student's training. By doing so, the teacher provides the ideal conditions whereby the student can become more present and conscious of what needs to be changed within him/herself. This supports what Patanjali refers to as *svadhyaya* or "self-study."

I have come to believe that life itself provides whatever experiences each soul needs to recognize the sharp corner's of one's ego, and that therefore the most effective process is to concentrate on *svadhyaya* or "self-study." This includes self-observation, using a journal as a tool, noticing one's habitual, repetitive reactions, which indicate samskaras, or habit patterns, and systematically weakening them by what Patanjali refers to as "opposite doing." *Svadhyaya* also includes regular study of the Self, through deep meditation, becoming aware of what is aware, and the study of sacred texts. These remind us of the underlying reality behind the apparent dramas of our lives.

I have also come to believe that at no matter what level we are on our spiritual path, our fellow travellers, whether they are teachers, fellow students, friends or family members, are the best mirrors we can look into, to see our ego, and its manifestations. So seeing, we can detach from the attachments and aversions, which our social relationships reveal. Such relationships are most revealing when we are with persons who are concentrating themselves on being aware and processing their own ego manifestations. This is the greatest insurance against what often happens when a "spiritual" person lives alone, and begins to believe that he is almost perfect.

So, "holy madness" is not inevitable. If sanity is defined as the ability to adjust to change, then those who are the sanest are those who can be in the world but not be disturbed by it. As Ramana Maharshi responded when someone asked him to describe his state of enlightenment: "Now, nothing can disturb me anymore." Today, our modern world is continuously changing, and the challenges which it presents, provide us with all that we need to confront and transcend the ego's attachments and aversions. May we all see the unchanging reality, the supreme truth in the midst of change, established in the perspective of our soul. May we all find the sacred, the holy, in the midst of the madness of the modern world.

7. How do we know whether we are progressing spiritually?

How do we know whether we are progressing spiritually? This is an important question that every spiritual aspirant asks himself or herself at one time or another. There is no easy answer. Because the spiritual path is progressive and because the spirit has no form, it is difficult to measure. So, before defining progress, let us define what we mean by "spiritual."

In Yoga, we talk about the human dilemma of egoism, of identifying with the body and mind. We refer to five bodies: the physical body (*anna maya kosha*, literally, the food body), the vital body (*prana maya kosha*, which animates the physical, and is the seat of emotions), the mental body (*mano maya kosha*, including subconscious, memory, five senses, recognition faculties), the intellectual body (*vinjnana maya kosha*, including our reasoning faculties), and the spiritual body (*ananda maya kosha*, literally, the bliss body, or soul, which is pure consciousness, the Witness). Ordinarily, because of egoism, one thinks and acts with the belief that "I" am the body, or "I" am my emotions, or "I" am my memories or ideas. For example, one says: "I" am cold; or "I" am angry; or "I" am married to so and so; "I" am "Jane Doe," or "I" am a Republican. Yet, a month later, one might identify with their opposites: "I" am hot; "I" am content; "I" am divorced; "I" have a new legal name: "Jane Smith;" and I switched parties, and now "I" am a Democrat. Obviously, we cannot be both opposites; we can only be what is....always. Yet, the power of egoism is so strong, that we constantly forget who we truly are: pure being and consciousness.

Therefore "spiritual progress" must involve a progressive identification with the *ananda maya kosha* or spiritual body, and a progressive letting go of the false identification with the physical, emotional, mental and intellectual bodies or dimensions of existence. This is a progressive purification from egoism, whose manifestations include: desire, anger, greed, pride, infatuation, and malice. In the beginning, and for a long time, this purification involves making efforts to respect ethical, moral and religious injunctions, for example, not harming, not stealing, and not lusting. These efforts enable one to gradually find an inner balance, based upon love, contentment, and acceptance. To use a modern analogy, the ego has us sitting too close to the television program of our life. Consequently, we are so absorbed in the drama that we forget who we truly are. Purifying ourselves of lust, greed, and anger, enables us to move back and away from the television screen, far enough that we begin to see that we are not the television program, with all the dramas in our life; we are its observer or Witness. What remains to be done, through spiritual practices like

MAKING OUR LIFE OUR YOGA

meditation, is to stand back further, and develop progressively a higher perspective on ourselves.

Ultimately, as we will see at the end of this article, once the state of Self-realization is mastered, it begins to descend into the intellectual, mental, vital and physical bodies, transforming them. Our spiritual development need not be "up and out" of this world. It can, as we will see involve an integrated development of all five planes of existence.

Initially, however, we are progressing spiritually to the extent that we identify increasingly with that part of us which is pure consciousness, or the Witness. This is known as Self-realization. This occurs in the following stages:

1. The development of calmness. Calmness is not the absence of thoughts, but being present with them. So, as we progress in this initial stage, we gradually replace the habit of reacting in habitual manners, for example with anger or anxiety, with a calm presence. The stain of mental delusion, known as *maya*, is weakened gradually by cultivating calmness. All of the practices of Yoga, including postures, systematic breathing, mantras, meditation and devotional activities help us in this stage to diminish agitation and unnecessary activity (*rajas*) and to weaken inertia, doubt and laziness (*tamas*) with quiet, calm, equanimity (sattva). This brings presence, or beingness (*sat*). By practicing detachment, we begin to let go of our need to be absorbed in the experiences.

2. The development of the Witness, or Chit, pure consciousness. We adopt a new perspective, by keeping part of our awareness standing back, observing. The Witness does not do or think anything. It simply watches actions happening or thoughts or emotions or sensations coming and going. Part of our consciousness is involved in the activities, part is standing back passively. We begin this stage with the effort to practice being a continuous witness, for relatively short periods or from the beginning to the end of an activity. This is possible especially while doing routine activities, not requiring much concentration, or for which we are conditioned to doing. Subsequently, it enters even activities which are challenging, or experienced for the first time, for example, when we have an accident, and fall. This perspective becomes more and more effortless, and integrated with daily life activities.

3. "I am not the Doer." As our Witness consciousness develops we no longer feel that we are doing anything, because we no longer identify

with the body and mental movements. Rather, we feel that we are only an observer and that our body and mind is an instrument. Part of our consciousness is involved in doing things, whether it be walking, talking, working, eating, etc., but now part of our consciousness stands back. It does nothing. It remains in a passive state of non-judgmental attention. One feels as if one is an instrument, and that the Divine does everything. One feels that there is "no doer" within. Yet everything gets done. One enjoys the play of events, their synchronicity, and consequences. One appreciates more and more how actions, words, and thoughts bring about consequences, or karma, and how this law can be applied to bring happiness rather than suffering to others. With this new expanded sense of Self, one feels that the needs of others are one's own. One expresses one's love for others, helping them to find happiness.

4. "I am That I am" In deep meditation we become aware of what is aware. Consciousness itself becomes the object. We feel that "I am in everything" and "Everything is in me." Later, and gradually this realization of the Self begins to permeate our waking daily activities. God realization comes as this stage deepens. Saints and mystics from all spiritual traditions have attempted to describe this, but words generally fail them. In fact, the more one tries to describe it, the further from it one goes, because describing it, or even thinking about it, reduces it to a set of ideas. As "IT" transcends all names and forms, permeates everything and is infinite and eternal, all else pales in significance. Silence is therefore the preferred medium of instruction for those who truly know "IT". As Swami Rama Tirtha, the first Yogi to bring Yoga to America, at the end of the 19th century, put it cogently: "A God defined, is a God confined. What this is all about can't be talked about, and it can't be whistled either."

The above stages are not a straight line. We zig-zag through them frequently because of the unstable nature of the mind, and our habitual habits (samskaras), karma, maya and the action of the gunas. But in general, this is the direction of our movement if we are progressing spiritually. Our identification with the body, emotions and mental movements weakens and is replaced with an identification with That, which is beyond names and forms, which is the Self, Pure consciousness, and which is ultimately Divine.

Progressive conceptions and perspectives of God

Our conception of God, or a Supreme Being, will also develop progressively, through stages, which are parallel to the above stages of spiritual development. From something which is "out there" to what is "inside me." It is instructive to analyze how we think about God, and what we identify with, both evolve as we progress on the spiritual path. By doing so we can avoid getting stuck at a lower stage. Theologians have categorized religion's several progressive conceptions of God. Each religion or cultural group assumes that their conception of God is the only correct one. It is evident that one's conception of God is limited by one's education, understanding of nature, personal experience, imagination, desires and fears. The human situation is projected upon one's conception of God. The following illustrates this.

Level one: God is my ally. I am the physical body.

The belief in a supreme being comes when one becomes aware of fear, and the greatest fear is that of death. Primitive man sought to overcome fears by attributing events in nature to supernatural sources. To allay these fears, primitive man offered sacrifices, in the hope that these would appease angry spirits, which were responsible for thunder, flood, drought, war, disease, and death. Supernatural beings, whether malevolent or benevolent could be foes or allies, in early polytheistic religions. Believers sought protection from deities and goddesses, to ward off evil, malevolent forces, and consequent suffering. Supernatural forces could be capricious, even vengeful. Life was short, brutish, and survival was the biggest issue, so above all, protection was needed. In this stage, one identifies primarily with one's physical body, and survival is the primary issue. If I am only the body, then evil is what threatens my survival. Good is what brings safety, food and shelter. So, I pray to a God, who as an ally provides to me what I need to survive. The stain of ignorance as to one's true identity, and consequently, egoism is deeply ingrained in the physical body.

Level two: God is omnipotent. I am the mind and personality.

Once society becomes stable, and survival is not a primary issue, humans sought to form laws to govern their social behavior. They attributed the authority for their laws to an "Almighty" God. Here, God is the source of all power and authority. Those who acquire power, do so, moreover because God has given it to them. Chieftains become kings, judges become priests. But power becomes intoxicating, because the more one acquires it, the more one's desires seek it. The individual, now freed from survival issues, identifies with the mind and vital's desires. The ego, the habit of identifying with the body and mind, now encompasses a nearly unlimited range of possibilities, as desires expand. One competes with others. One is selfish. With power one seeks to accomplish, to dominate others, to fulfill one's ambitions. One does so, however, while trying to respect the laws which are given by God, fearing punishment, if transgressed. Religious dogma and institutions are elaborated in response to an expanding intellectual curiosity, while seeking to control human nature, and keep it subordinate to those who rule. Science develops and challenges religion. Religions clash. Cultures clash. Political and religious institutions become allied. One even prays to God to defeat one's enemies or convert others whose beliefs differ from one's own. It is "us" against "them."

Level 3: God is Stillness: "Be Still and know that I am God." I witness.

Many individuals reach this stage when, for one reason or another, they discover an inner being, which is behind the movements of the body, senses and mind. It may be a spontaneous spiritual experience, in which one transcends; it may be the result of practicing a formal meditation exercise; it may occur as a result of an intense physical experience which involves pain, or great concentration in which one detaches from the ordinary mental state. As a result, one begins to realize that one's previous conceptions of God were just conceptions, that is, one begins to realize that one has up to now created a God to serve one's own egoistic needs, with all of its fears and desires. One realizes that one's view of the world "out there" is distorted by one's own likings and dislikings. But in level 3, one finds peace, and so God is peace. One realizes the truth of the Psalms: "Be Still and know that I am God." One realizes that it is only by developing the inner perspective of one's true Self, a Witness consciousness, that one can overcome the turmoil of the outer world. In the Stillness of the mind, one discovers pure consciousness. It is like the light in the room, which up until now, was ignored, as one was preoccupied with what was reflected by the light, the contents of the room. In the beginning, there is a tension between one's inner and outer life, which may result in one rejecting the latter.

As this stage progresses, one seeks to cultivate calm, meditative awareness throughout all of the moments of one's life. One does not reject the world. In the words of Jesus, one is in the world, but not of it. One replaces thinking about God, that is, concepts, with a new witness perspective, wherein one is no longer absorbed in thoughts, but at peace with a quiet mind. In effect, one rises above the mental movements, into "the light of consciousness." Words cannot express. Poetry can point to it. "It is a peace which passeth all understanding," mentioned by the mystics and seers of all spiritual traditions. At this level, religion and every other intellectual system is submerged into spirituality.

Level 4: God is Wise. I listen, I know

Having gone beyond the primary issues of fear and desire, and having found inner peace, one realizes that God loves me, that he forgives me, that he understands. Therefore, he is wise. God is all knowing, and so, by listening to God, I also know. I listen to him, by being calm, receptive and allowing my intuition to speak. I begin to identify with the one who knows, not because I learned something in school, but because I just know. I understand more and more, spontaneously, whenever I focus on what it is I need to know. Things become clear. I see the underlying truth behind everything, and wisdom comes to me. I can distinguish what is permanent from what is impermanent, what brings joy from what brings suffering, and Who I Am, truly, the eternal soul, pure consciousness. One's concern is no longer with following the rules, and avoiding what is painful, particular in the "outer" world of turmoil, however, as in previous levels. One turns towards transcendental loving God, with full confidence, and cherishing That in one's heart constantly, one feels loved, purified, and guided by the Lord intuitively. At the end of this stage, one feels completely innocent, having let go of all notions of right and wrong, guilt and pride. One identifies with others, loves them and helps them to find happiness.

Level 5: God is my co-creator. I create

At this level of spiritual development, one realizes that one has the power and the responsibility to create one's life. One goes beyond the ordinary state of "dreaming with one's open," to that of a visionary. One becomes a visionary. One remains faithful to one's dreams, the dreams which one knows are in alignment with one's path of wisdom and Self-realization. The Lord is no longer distant, and one feels that one is a "co-creator" with the Lord. The Lord gives graciously. The Lord inspires. When one sets one's intention to make something happen, consequently, the universe conspires to support one in bringing about its fulfillment. One may have to work hard for its accomplishment, but one feels that one is not the doer, just an instrument. One is patient about the outcome, trusting that the universe will take care of it. One abides in the present moment and things get done as one does whatever is needed. One aligns oneself more and more with the will of the Lord, however, as one purifies the ego's needs and preferences. Whatever the result, one feels blessed.

Level 6: God is a wonder. I am effulgent self-awareness

With God as one's co-creator, one begins to see the world as a miracle of creation, and our lives are a playground. Miracles abound. God is "ever-new joy," in the words of Yogananda, so awesome is every moment, every event. One sees the Lord as that which is beyond all causation, unaffected by creation, the light of consciousness. One realizes that at one's own deepest Self is the same: effulgent self-awareness. Light is a metaphor for consciousness, but it is also what mystics experience in the depths of their soul. The Lord is beyond time, beyond space, unlimited by anything. At this level, the grace of the Lord brings many wondrous occurrences. One finds sacredness in the mundane. One sees with the eyes of the mystic, the Presence of the Lord everywhere. Grace, unlike karma, is undeserved, and does not depend upon whether our actions are good or bad; it is the response of the Lord to one's call to unite with That which is beyond names and forms, to give up the duality of liking and disliking, having and losing, success and failure, fame and shame. One recognizes that the ego's game, with all of its desire is a huge trap, and one surrenders to the Lord, not just mentally, but consciously. One seeks liberation from the ego's games. One becomes absorbed in that which is beyond the mental movement, their fundamental source, the light of consciousness.

Level 7: God is Absolute Being Consciousness and Bliss. "I am"

Having escaped the duality of the mind, one arrives at the non-dual state of *sat chit ananda*, or absolute being, consciousness and bliss. This state is unconditional, in that it depends upon nothing. It simply is, and one realizes that "That I am." One becomes nothing special; one experiences nothing special. For specialness implies being apart, and at this level one has transcended the pairs of opposites, and realized one's unity with everything. At this level, which theologians would classify as *monism*, there is only One. In theism, there is the soul and the Lord, and they are separate. From the perspective of *monism*, there is only One.

That One, is infinite, unchanging, eternal, beyond description, the source of everything. One accesses That when in the deepest states of meditation, the mind becomes silent, yet consciousness expands. When Moses asked God "Who are you?" when God spoke to him through the burning bush, the Lord replied "I am that I am." This expresses both the ultimate objective and subjective states of existence, "I" the subject, and "That" the object. It is not a void. It is the source of everything; it is supreme intelligence itself. Being here now then becomes the only way to go! Being, not doing becomes the vehicle and destination. Being present, no matter what the drama, brings awareness, and awareness brings bliss: "*sat chit ananda.*" And you can no longer answer the question "Who are you?" except with a reply that "I am." Any other reply is seen to be a case of mistaken identity, the ego's game. One's old habitual tendencies, preferences and dislikes fade into the background, and the feeling of "I am" rules. There is no more "other." There is no more special status, no "master" no "Guru" no "devotee," no "disciple." There is only One. This realization, known as *samadhi*, in Yoga, comes during deep meditative experiences, and for many years, can be elusive, because one is ordinarily so conditioned to identify with memories, the body and the mind. But by returning repeatedly to this state, the stains of ignorance, egoism, delusion and karma gradually fades in the effulgent bleach of Self-realization. One no longer seeks special experiences, nor to be special. Because specialness creates separation, and when one becomes one with everything, there is no other.

Transformation

Saints of all spiritual traditions who reach this state find that it is so fulfilling that the desire to remain in this world gradually fades, along with all other desires. The body, with all of its needs, continues to be a distraction, and so, even advanced saints, who have reached this seventh state, depart from this world without complaint, either bound for heaven or in quest of liberation from the round of birth and rebirth.

However, in China, Tibet and India, there exists an ancient tradition of spiritual adepts who have envisioned that spiritual development does not end in the spiritual plane of existence, as described in the seventh stage above. Realizing that the Lord is Here, their surrender to the Lord went beyond surrendering their soul to the Lord, in the spiritual dimension. Surrendering their intellect, the desire to know, they became sages, capable of profound knowledge on any subject they turned their minds to. Such knowledge came not in the usual way, through study or empirical research, but by intuitively becoming one with the object of interest. This insightful knowledge, expressed the most profound of truths, often defying expression, a product of supreme intelligence in deep states of concentration and cognitive absorption, known as samadhi.

Surrendering further, at the level of the mind, such adepts became "siddhas," or one's who could manifest latent powers, such as clairvoyance, prophecy, and clairaudience. Surrendering themselves at the level of the vital, maha siddhas, or great, and perfect adepts, manifested still greater powers, such as levitation, materialization of objects, dematerialization of themselves, control over nature, control over events. Surrendering at the level of the physical, even the cells gave up their limited agenda of reproduction, and became intimately connected to the will and consciousness of the adept. The body became invulnerable, deathless, no longer subject to the laws of nature. Such a progressive surrender to the Lord expresses not an aspiration for liberation from this world of suffering, but as one's aspiration to allow the Lord to manifest through oneself at all levels of existence, in all five bodies, spiritual, intellectual, mental, vital and physical. No longer seeing a division between matter and spirit, but only spirit, that all is Divine, such Siddhas, are the leading edge of humanity's evolution. For them, to realize God in a diseased body is not perfection. They have fulfilled the injunction of Jesus to his disciples to "Be ye perfect, even as your Father in heaven is perfect."

8. The Yoga of the 21st Century

The French philosopher, André Malraux, predicted that "the next century will be spiritual or it will not be at all." While the immediate threat of nuclear self-destruction has receded with the end of the Cold War, the real battle continues to be waged in the hearts and minds of billions of people in the world today. What some modern thinkers have termed "deep ecology" refers to the ancient yogic recognition of the interrelationship between our spirit, mind, body and environment.

In the past, many looked upon yoga with suspicion, perhaps because it came from an exotic foreign culture. However, today, it is becoming a household word, all around the world. In the USA alone, a recent survey by Roper Associates estimated that more than 6 million persons are practicing it. That is about 5 percent of the adult population! While there are still 95 percent who are not, what is significant is the effect that this 5 percent can have on their neighbors. While most yoga practitioners are still only practicing Hatha Yoga, and little or no meditation, there is a growing awareness that yoga is not just standing on your head, or stretching your body.

What are we to do, knowing this? The consensus among the participants of our recent International Gathering can be summarized in three phrases:

1. practice yogic sadhana

2. integrate yoga with work and family life;

3. inform others.

The practice of yogic sadhana is so important, not only for our personal well being and health, but for everyone around us. When we practice yoga, there is an immediate energetic effect on our environment and those with whom we come into contact. Peace, joy, awareness are all contagious!

Bringing yoga into work and family life means practicing equanimity during stressful periods, becoming aware of tension, using the breath as a monitor, and doing our work as karma yoga, skilfully, but unattached to the results. It means "being present" with others, especially those with whom we live and work, allowing our love and goodwill to radiate towards them. Yoga develops the art of being a good listener.

Informing others means educating them as to what yoga is, its benefits, and clarifying frequent misconceptions. That requires one to study both ancient and modern sources, to sharpen ones understanding and ability to communicate yoga's truths. It includes being sensitive to cultural differences, and if possible, showing them how yoga really works, to release tension, get a good night's sleep, find a new vibrant source of energy, health and inner calm. It could also involve sharing favorite books on yoga with friends and acquaintances, writing articles for magazines or the web, giving talks or classes in the postures or beginning meditation or the path of yoga. It is time for yoga to recognize itself as a social movement, wherein its practitioners reach out to others and share the best of themselves.

We are entering a new era where yoga will not only be a household word, but a powerful current leading our civilization to great heights.

9. Tapas: Voluntary Self-Challenge

As a young *brahmacharya* in the early 1970's my teacher often challenged me with requests that I make specific vows. These included vows of silence one day per week, vows of fasting one day per week, practice of a specific technique every day for 48 days, weekly recitation of the Kriya Yoga Pledge before beginning silence, a vow of celibacy, and vegetarianism, repetition of mantras every day for a minimum number of times, practice of yogic sadhana eight hours per day, and more general vows of dedication to the overall practice of Babaji's Kriya Yoga. He also challenged me to practice Yoga for 24 hours without stopping, referring to this as "*tapas.*" These things I did regularly during the 18 years I spent under his tutelage. I have written about these austerities and experiences in "How I became a disciple." Why did I do such things, you may ask?

Tapas and self-purification

The great questions of life "Who am I?" "How can I know God?" "How can I find lasting happiness in a world of suffering?" can only be answered, according to the great spiritual traditions, by a process of purification. As humans, we are deeply flawed because of our ignorance of the Self and because of egoism, which causes us to identify with the body and the mind. Our attachments and aversions cause us further suffering. Yoga offers a practical means for overcoming these human imperfections. While Yoga can be viewed from many different perspectives, one of the most useful ways of seeing it is as a complete system of self-purification. *Tapas* or austerity is the use of vows, will-power and endurance to purify oneself, by overcoming the limitations of our habit patterns. According to Patanjali, "By *tapas* (austerity) impurities of the body and senses are destroyed and perfection gained." (Yoga-Sutras I.43)

The word "*tapas*" literally means "heat" or "glow." The early name for a yogin, in the Vedas, the most ancient spiritual texts of India, was *tapasvin* or practioner of *tapas,* voluntary self-challenge. *Surya*, the name for the Lord in the Vedas, refers to the Solar Deity. According to the Vedas, *Surya* is the original practitioner of *tapas,* and so, is the originator of Yoga, known as *Hiranyagarbha* (Golden Womb or Sun). In the Bhagavad

Gita (4.1) the Sun, *Vivasvat* is referred to as the primordial teacher of Yoga. Ancient Yogins or *tapasvins* were sun-worshippers, and remnants of this archaic Yoga are still found in the Sun Salutation series common to all traditions of Hatha Yoga.

Patanjali tells us in Yoga-Sutra III.55 that enlightenment occurs when the mind becomes purified like a mirror, and is able to reflect the natural luminosity of the Self, pure consciousness: "In the sameness of purity between beingness and the Self, there is absolute freedom."

Tapas means "intense practice" or "austerity." It refers to any intense or prolonged practice for Self-realization, which involves overcoming the natural tendencies of the body, emotions or mind. Because of the resistance of the body, emotions or mind, heat or pain may develop as a biproduct, but this is never the objective. The objective is to overcome their dominance and absorption of our consciousness.

In Yoga-Sutra II.1, Patanjali defines Kriya Yoga as: "*tapas* (intense practice), *svadhyaya* (self-study) and *isvara-pranidhana* (devotion to the Lord.)" In Sutra I.13 he explains clearly what we are to practice: "In this context, the effort to abide in (the cessation of identification with the fluctuations of consciousness) is a constant practice."

The three components of tapas: intention, willpower, and endurance

Tapas begins with an intention or a vow to deny oneself some indulgence. It could involve anything: a physical pleasure, certain food, casual sex, television, or if sitting in meditation, making an unnecessary movement. When we fix our intention, we are setting our goal. We do this firmly, not with an expression of hope, or maybe in the future I will, but a clear message to one's subconscious that "I am" now doing this. For how long? That is to be determined by the vow or intention. For example: meditation for 30 minutes, 60 minutes, observing silence or fasting for one day, abstention from a particular food, beverage or pleasurable activity for one month.

The second and third components of tapas are willpower and endurance. As with an athlete, who develops his physical strength, the *tapasvin* develops his willpower gradually, by repeatedly and regularly exercising it. One begins with relatively short periods of postponing the satisfaction of a desire or aversion. It often involves standing back from any particular attachment or aversion, or any thought or feeling of "I am this feeling, sensation or thought" and letting it go. This is known as "*vairagya*" or "detachment." This requires effort and willpower, and consistent repetition for an extended period. The postponement gradually becomes longer, and finally one may let go of it altogether. However, the accomplished *tapasvin*, eventually reaches a stage of equanimity, wherein one may simply enjoy, whether the object of desire or aversion is present or not. So, intention, effort and endurance are the key elements of *tapas*.

In our pleasure seeking and consumerist lifestyle, such voluntary abstention and denial will strike the majority of persons as irrational and inconsistent with what is known today as "the good life." Such persons fail to recognize the delight, which lies within ourselves, waiting to be discovered when control is exercised over neurotic impulses of attachment and aversion. The mind constantly dwells upon desires and fears, but when one exercises a little dispassion towards these, they vanish like clouds in the sky.

The Bhagavad Gita (17.14-16) speaks of three kinds of *tapas*: austerity of body, speech and mind. Austerity of the body includes cleanliness, chastity, non-violence, courteous behavior, compassionate actions, and devotional activities. Austerity of speech includes speaking only what is truthful, helpful, and necessary, after reflection, giving no offence. It may include chanting of the Lord's name in devotional activities. Austerity of the mind includes silence, serenity, concentration, discrimination, and avoidance of unkind thoughts. These austerities cultivate uplifting emotions associated with love, gratitude, courage and acceptance.

Tapas should be done without expectation of reward and with faith in the process of Yoga. In this way one develops equanimity, which is the pre-requisite for enlightenment. Whether there is success or failure, loss or gain, whether it is comfortable or uncomfortable, hot or cold, whether one is rested or tired, one maintains a calm acceptance of what is, in the present moment. One goes beyond duality to unity.

By cultivating *tapas*, one develops great energy and willpower, which enables one to master one's life, and overcome all obstacles. One develops the light of supramental consciousness. One becomes radiant like the sun, not only in the subtle bodies, but ultimately even in the physical. One becomes a source of light, warmth and love for everyone.

10. Samadhi

When a person begins his or her study of Yoga they usually have little or no idea of what are its ultimate objectives. In the contemporary world of Yoga, Yoga has become like a supermarket: you can find whatever you are looking for in it. One's current needs, whether they are physical, emotional, mental, intellectual or spiritual tend to motivate the student. Today, most often, students are looking for a way to control the effects of stress or to find some peace of mind. It is generally a "quick fix" approach, in which there is a temporary relief from the uncomfortable symptoms of the stress and strain of life.

Occasionally, one hears someone speak of higher "spiritual" goals, such as *"Samadhi"* or "Self-realization" or "enlightenment." But they are usually described in such a way as to lead the average student to believe that it practically impossible "to attain" such exalted states, so why even try? Descriptions of it, are therefore fuzzy at best, and absent at worst. But without a clear idea of what are the ultimate objectives of Yoga, the student of Yoga is bound to miss it. Even when they may have glimpses of it, the student may not recognize its value. Worse, the student may confuse some passing spiritual experience as something worth holding onto or repeating.

"Samadhi is not what you think"

This statement is quite literally true, because *"samadhi"* is what you don't think; it involves silence of the mind. That is why it also true that the more you talk about *samadhi*, the further from it you go. There is a saying: "Those who talk about *samadhi* don't know it, and those who know don't talk about it." It is the space between thoughts. It is not an object, and it cannot be understood. It transcends all forms and ideas. It is therefore not an experience, and it only when you are prepared to experience nothing special and to be nothing special, that you may realize *samadhi*. It is the subject, not an object. While you can never know *samadhi*, it is possible to be in it, when your consciousness becomes aware of what is aware: this is what is meant by the definition, "cognitive absorption." One's consciousness becomes absorbed in itself. In *samadhi*, one ceases to identify with the body, the emotions, and the thoughts. Egoism is temporarily suspended.

Samadhi generally comes and goes as the resistance of one's human nature repeatedly pulls one back into ordinary consciousness. This occurs until one has purified the *samskaras*, or subconscious habits sufficiently, and cultivated a high degree of equilibrium, physically, emotionally and then mentally. It is only after many years of repeatedly entering into the lower stages of samadhi, known as *samprajnata samadhi*, that the higher level, *asamprajnata*, or *nirvikalpa samadhi* enables one to become enlightened. Enlightenment can be defined as a continuous state of *samadhi* or Self-realization. Even this is not the final attainment however. Generally limited to the spiritual plane, the enlightened person or saint, may still possess a diseased body or neurotic mind. It is only when and if they surrender these completely to the Divine that one becomes progressively a sage, a siddha and a maha-siddha.

In the third initiation one learns several Kriyas which enable one to go into the *samadhi* states fairly easily. One's sadhana really begins here, however, as one must learn to stabilize the samadhi state continuously, rather than intermittently.

Finding authentic guidance to *samadhi*

Another problem is that in the contemporary world, Yoga and "personal growth" has become a big business, whether it be through books or seminars, and there are a lot of competing alternative approaches, mostly untested and of recent origin. How is the student to yoga to decide what is authentic? Which path will lead him to the ultimate objectives of Yoga? What are the ultimate objectives?

To answer these questions, it is useful to return to the oldest authoritative sources, such as the *Yoga-sutras* of Patanjali and the *Thirumandiram* by Thirumoolar. Patanjali defines the ultimate objective of Yoga as "*samadhi*," "cognitive absorption." In aphorism I.17 he describes the first level of *samadhi*: "*samprajnata*:" "Object-oriented cognitive absorption is accompanied by observation, reflecting, rejoicing and pure I-am-ness." In ordinary physical consciousness, our awareness is absorbed by objects of attention through the five senses. In day dreaming or thinking our consciousness is absorbed by thoughts, memories and emotions. In both of these, we are unaware of "that which is aware." In "cognitive absorption" we become "conscious of what is conscious," the Seer, the pure subject. Objects of attention are in the background. The Self or Seer comes to the foreground of our awareness. We identify with the Seer, rather than with the thoughts or sensations or emotions.

In ordinary consciousness, Patanjali tells us in verse I.6 that we identify with the five types of *"vrittis"* or modifications arising within consciousness: "right knowledge, misconception, verbal delusion, sleep and memory."

"Samprajnata Samadhi"

In *"samprajnata"* or distinguished cognitive absorption, there are four accompaniments. They are not mere "mental" modifications or *"vrittis,"* but inspired products of this fusion between subject and object. Unlike the higher samadhi *"asamprajnata"* samadhi, here there are material or subtle objects as supports, or points of departure. These supports may be any of the forms of Nature, including the most sublime levels of transcendental existence.

Here it is appropriate to first explain some of the oldest concepts in Indian metaphysical thought: the terms *"prakriti"* (Nature) and *"purusha"* (Self) mentioned in verses I.16 and I.24. Prakriti is everything besides the Self and includes the entire cosmos from the material to the psychic levels. Unlike the Self (I am...), which is purely subjective, *prakriti* is objective reality, that which is observed by the Self. It is Real, however transitory it may be. Purusha, the Self, is pure subject, at the core of consciousness. It illuminates the consciousness. Without it, the mind and psyche would have no conscious activity, just as a light bulb without invisible electricity would radiate no light. Prakriti exists as Nature in its transcendental, undefined state and its multi-form, differentiated manifestations.

To know *purusha* one must first understand *prakriti*. The first step comes by contemplating nature in its various manifestations:

1. *Vitarka* = Observation and analysis of material Nature, down to its elemental characteristics.

"Savitarka" samadhi occurs when the mind is focused on an object in Nature.

We can realize this by means of "Tradak Kriyas," concentration on and absorption in material objects, or the Dhyana Kriyas involving the five subtle elements, the *"jnana indriyas."*

2. V*icara* = Reflection on subtle nature experiencing the truth of abstractions, without reference to material observation.

"Savicara" samadhi occurs when the mind is focused on an abstraction.

We can realize this by means of the Dhyana Kriyas involving abstract concepts such as "Truth," "Love," "Wisdom."

3. Ananda = Pure joy. Rejoicing, which is independent of outer circumstances, is an accompaniment of cognitive absorption.

"*Sananda*" samadhi occurs when joy itself is the only object without any form or abstraction.

The practice of "Nityananda Kriya" taught in Babaji's Kriya Yoga Second and Third Level Initiations helps one to become aware of this.

4. *Asmita* = I-am-ness. This is pure subjectivity.

"*Sa-asmita*" samadhi occurs when we are only aware of "I am;" however the samskaras, or subconscious tendencies are still buried in a seed form in the mind, and may manifest given a stimulus.

By practicing the various "Samadhi Kriyas" taught in Babaji's Kriya Yoga Third level Initiation, going inward from the gross to the most subtle levels, one can separate *purusha* from *prakriti*, and realize these four accompaniments of the first level of samadhi.

"Asamprajnata Samadhi"

In verse I.18 Patanjali tells us: "By constant practice of the thought of detachment (towards mental modifications) only the thought of detachment itself remains as a residual subconscious impression. This is the other samadhi "*asamprajnata Samadhi*" (non-distinguished) (which follows) the previous ("*samprajnata*"). Here there are no longer objective supports. After understanding "*prakrit,*" nature in its four manifestations "*prajnata*" - object oriented cognitive absorption. Their cessation occurs only after constant and prolonged practice of detachment through various methods. "*Asamprajnata* (non-distinguished) *samadhi*" follows *samprajnata samadhi* and becomes possible only with a moment to moment practice of detachment and Self-awareness for many years. Supreme detachment is therefore the means to attain it, because it cannot be attained when an object is the basis of concentration. Only the latent impression of detachment itself remains.

In verse I.20 Patanjali tells us: "To the others, this *asamprajnata samadhi* is preceded by faith, memory, cognitive absorption and discernment." In contrast to those yogis referred to in the previous verse that leave the physical body before reaching *asamprajnata samadhi*, those who do reach it, do so by developing the following:

sraddha = Implicit faith in Yoga, with confidence in one's capacity, one's sadhana or methods, and one's preceptor.

virya = Energy or enthusiasm arises from such faith and produces intense devotion wherein the emotions also support one's practice.

smriti = Memory; where one remembers the path constantly, the lessons learned, so as not to fall back into a worldly perspective; one remains attentive;

samadhi = One regularly cultivates the experience of cognitive absorption. Though it is not constant due to the fluctuations of the mind and distractions, it develops by means of yogic sadhana.

prajna = Discernment; insight. By vigilant Self-awareness, moment to moment, one receives insights and guidance through the events of life.

Spiritual energy and strength bring attentiveness and vigilance. One remembers the path constantly, and the lessons learned so as not to fall back into worldly perspectives. This memory brings contemplation uninterrupted.

Such continuous contemplation or *samadhi* brings discernment between the Real Self and non-real.

"Asamprajnata Samadhi" may come as an eventual consequence of repeated experiences of *"samprajnata Samadhi,"* as the subconscious tendencies gradually dissolve. However, it may also come as a result of the student cultivating certain positive tendencies, enumerated in the verse such as faith, enthusiasm, vigilance, discernment and contemplation. These will create the ideal conditions by which old tendencies can be dissolved.

"To the keen and intense practitioner this (samadhi) is near." verse I.21

One may have glimpses of *samadhi*, the experience of the Self, in which one's mind concentrates inwardly, and one is filled with absolute bliss, but the real challenge is for this to become prolonged and stable. To do so, one needs to practice with intense or enthusiastic devotion, to cultivate the witness consciousness and to consistently turn the mind and senses inward, away from the tendencies towards dispersion. When concentration and witness awareness become spontaneous and continuous, this is known as intense practice (*tivrasamavega*).

Whenever we gain a glimpse of *samadhi* in our inner being, we will be wise to carry it into our outer life as well. It says in the Shiva Sutras, "the bliss of the world is the bliss of *samadhi*."

"The difference in time necessary (for *samadhi*) further depends on whether the practice is mild, medium, or intense." - verse I.22

A mild practice is uneven, sporadic, full of doubts, ups and downs, full of distractions, which carry one away. A medium practice has periods of intensity and devotion, alternating with periods of forgetfulness, distractions, indulgences in negative thinking and habits. An intense practice is characterized by a constant determination to remember the Self and to maintain equanimity through success, and failure, pleasure and pain, growing in love, confidence, patience and sympathy for others. It becomes intense when we worship our chosen form of God, or try to see the Divinity pervading everything, to go beyond our desires, which rise up. No matter the intensity of the events or circumstances, no matter how great the *maya*, or play of the illusion-filled drama, we continue to see the Divinity throughout.

To develop an intense practice, get immersed in doing the Yoga. Take a step forward every day. See everything as part of the Divine Plan, unfolding perfectly for your evolution. See nothing as outside of that Divine Plan, or contrary to it. With this in mind be persistent and consistent.

11. Kaivalyam: Absolute Freedom

What is the ultimate goal of Yoga? In the fourth and final *pada* (chapter) of the Yoga-Sutras, Patanjali elaborates on this question, and defines it as: *kaivalyam*. Most translators and commentators have translated this term as "Aloneness," particularly those who have emphasized Patanjali's philosophical dualism. They have concluded that the final goal of the realized soul is departure from the physical plane. Divorce between the spirit and the flesh again, which is so often repeated in spiritual literature. While Patanjali's Kriya Yoga, is based upon the *Samkhya* philosophy, as exemplified by *purusha (*consciousness, the Self, the Seer, the subject) versus *prakriti* (Nature, the Seen, the object) in my book, *The Kriya Yoga Sutras of Patanjali and the Siddhas*, I have shown the influence of Tantra, in general, and Siddhantha in particular, on Patanjali's philosophy and theology. Based upon this new perspective, another meaning of the word "*kaivalyam*" as "Absolute Freedom" is more precise.

As *kaivalyam* is the goal of Classical Yoga, it is important to have a clear understanding of the meaning of this term. Most commentators, such as the noted scholar, Dr. Georg Feuerstein, have concluded rather bleakly that the goal of "Aloneness" as described by Patanjali, requires that one leave behind this world when one reaches the highest state of "non-distinguished cognitive absorption," (Sutra I.18) known as *asamprajnata samadhi*.

This conclusion is perhaps rooted in the bias against Nature, and especially "human nature," which seems to pervade spiritual traditions in general, and enunciate traditions in particular. In this bias, there is the assumption that the laws of Nature are immutable, and that therefore the only way around them, so to speak, is to leave this world behind. This ignores the great potential for the Self-realized soul to transform its human vehicle, including the intellectual, mental, vital and even the physical bodies. The Yoga Siddhas, and more recently Sri Aurobindo and contemporary writers such as Ken Wilbur have however, affirmed our potential for such a transformation of our human nature on a collective scale. But there are many older sources in the literature of the Yoga Siddhas. Unfortunately, until recently, these sources have been largely ignored outside of very limited circles of initiates.

At the beginning of the Yoga-Sutras, (I.3) Patanjali informs us of this when he says: "The Seer abides in his own true form (*svarupa)*." That is, the individual soul or *jiva,* assumes by expansion, its true nature or form, Siva, the Supreme Consciousness. The perfection of cognitive absorption, in its progressive stages, as described by Patanjali and the Siddhas brings about a radical transformation at many levels. The ordinary human nature, previously motivated only by the constituent forces of nature (the *gunas)* is replaced by a higher nature (*svarupa*) according to Patanjali in the fourth *pada*. (see IV.34). The term *svarupa* means literally "ones own true form or nature." Tirumular and other siddhas have referred often to *svarupa* as "self-illuminating manifestness."

In verse II.25 Patanjali defines *kaivalyam* as follows: "Without this ignorance (*avidya*) no such union (*samyoga*) occurs. This is the absolute freedom (*kaivalyam*) from the Seen." Patanjali defines "*avidya*" in verse II.5 as "ignorance." There he states "Ignorance is seeing the impermanent as permanent, the impure as pure, the painful as pleasurable and the non-Self as the Self." In verse II.17 Patanjali informs us of *samyoga*, saying: "The cause (of suffering) to be eliminated is (*samyoga*) the union of Seer and the Seen." *Samyoga* may be understood as that ordinary state of human consciousness where the Self is identified with the objects of its experience: this is what is meant by "the union of Seer and the Seen." For example, when we say, "I am tired," or "I am concerned." Or "I want that," we are manifesting the state of *samyoga,* the union of the Seer and the Seen.

In the fourth pada, verse 27, Patanjali informs us that the method to free ourselves from this state of *samyoga* is to continue to detach from the false identification with the *vrittis* or fluctuations arising within consciousness and their attendant *klesas* or afflictions. This method is explained in sutra I.12: "By constant practice and with detachment (arises) the cessation (of identifying with the fluctuations of consciousness)." And in verse II.26 he says: "Uninterrupted discriminative discernment is the method for its removal."

The term *Siddhantha* means the final end of perfection or accomplishment for the Saivite. A *siddha* is one who manifests *siddhi* or perfection or special powers. "I am the Supreme one" says the *Vedantin*. "I shall become the Supreme One" says the *Siddhantin*. While *kaivalya* refers to the final attainments, it also marks the beginning of unlimited possibilities. But *kaivalyam* understood as a beginning of "absolute freedom" is synonymous with the state of a *Siddha*, who has allowed the Supreme Being to descend within himself or herself at all levels, in complete surrender. This brings about an integrated development at all levels, not simply a vertical ascent out of the world, as in most spiritual traditions. Only such an all-encompassing transformation merits recognition with the term "perfection." To be spiritually awakened in a diseased body, and a disturbed mind and vital, is not perfection. Whether a Siddha continues to remain on the physical plane is unimportant. If he or she does, it is only to be instrumental in the awakening and transformation of the human race. If they depart, it is not because they are forced to do so, due to a degeneration of the human organism. And unlike the *bodhisattva* vow in Buddhism, where one promises to return until all sentient beings reach final liberation, the Siddhantin is dedicated to the transformation of *this* world, which is not illusionary or without value. This world is intrinsically divine. It is our collective divine "edge" where the Lord, through us, realizes its greatest potential.

Thus the fourth *pada*, is not the final one. The final one is yet to be written by all of us, as we realize our evolutionary potential.

In Sutra IV.2, Patanjali informs us of not only the possibility, but the likelihood that the human species will evolve into something new, with as yet undreamed of possibilities:

"The transformation into another species (is due to) the vast possibilities inherent in Nature."

What the Siddhas attained individually can be a goal, or final attainment, for the rest of us, even collectively. The collective transformation of the human species is rarely referred to in spiritual liberation literature. Modern siddhas such as Sri Aurobindo and Ramalinga Swamigal have also provided much guidance. By following their example, and teachings, sincere students of Yoga may work towards such a goal of Absolute Freedom. They have shown us the path to such a complete surrender and transformation. Only then will our highest potential as human beings be realized. Only then will *kaivalyam,* absolute freedom, be realized.

12. Sadhana of Life

What is *sadhana*? The word *sadhana* comes from the Sanskrit root, *saad,* meaning "to go straight to a goal or aim; to accomplish; to master." *Sadhana* is a practice of remembrance of Self. It can be defined as a way of being, thinking and living that supports you in shifting your sense of self away from identification with your body, thoughts, emotions and personal history. *Sadhana* provides the experience of your awareness as the great Self.

Babaji's Kriya Yoga is "Action with Awareness" and it is a means of knowing the truth of our being. The Kriya Yoga *sadhana* is the daily practice of "Action with Awareness," which has enormous potential. All we have to do is to be willing participants. We have to be willing to align body, mind, heart and will with our soul. Kriya Yoga is not a pastime; it is a preoccupation with the Divine Self. The sadhana is not only a collection of 144 physical and mental exercises or spiritual practices. It is a way of life for our entire being. The mind, heart, soul and will align in aspiration of purification and perfection, in renunciation of ego's desires, in order to live to serve the Truth. By living to serve the Truth, our Yoga can offer us a larger and deeper life that is largely unaffected by the ups and downs of external circumstances. Kriya Yoga does not exclude life but asks us to embrace or at least to accept life and all its external manifestation, both pleasant and painful.

Kriya Yoga sees the external world as the outer manifestation of the Divine and uses it as one's personal field of sadhana.

It is through your life that you come to know the Truth of yourself. Your sadhana is contained within your life experiences. It is in this field of life experiences that you can most easily do your yogic work. It is through the experiences of your life that you are able to gain the most growth. Your soul draws its "juice," from life experiences. It is from this juice, the essence of the intense experiences of your outer being that you build a personality that is drawn towards the Divine Consciousness.

The map of Kriya Yoga suggests that we live in the world in order to attain self-observation, self-purification and realization of the Divine within us. It is not about liberation from the world but liberation within it. We do not need outer renunciation to bring us to the goal, for it is in the world that we are challenged by our attachments, aversions and cravings. True renunciation is purity; it is a renunciation in consciousness and a re-linquishment of ego, a dropping of the sense of "I" and "mine" from the heart. True renunciation is an inner state of conquering selfish thoughts, desires and even preferences while being in the world.

Unless you are confronted by your limited personality, how are you to have the truth revealed? In the world you develop attachments, aversions and cravings. The world exposes you to various temptations, suffering, lessons and guidance, whether or not you call yourself a yogi or claim a religious identity. Your sadhana is to reveal the truth about them. The world also offers you so much love to take delight in. It offers you so much beauty and wonder. Kriya Yoga sadhana can help you to see the love, wonder and beauty, which underlies every moment of life, even in the worst suffering.

Essentially there should be no real distinction between what you identify as your sadhana and what you define as your life. All your actions can be offered up to be transformed in the Divine Fire of Yoga. All your consciousness can be offered up to be transformed in that same Divine Fire. As a Kriya Yogi you assume the sincerest subservient role, so that your every action flows from the Divine within. To live in the world as a child of the Divine, this is the Awareness to acquire.

I would like to share with you a particular experience of mine, which made clear to me everything of which I have spoken of here. It occurred in a meeting I had with a Divine Child, who radiated spiritual beauty and wonder. Often outer beauty is a mix of vital power and magnetism, containing no spiritual power at all. Light of a vital nature is bright, white and cold. I had seen it before. But, spiritual beauty is charming and sweet and more powerfully transforming than physical beauty can ever be. Even with physical deformity, a spiritually beautiful person will strongly attract us …

Imagine a young man, about 20 years old, with a crippled body, paraplegic, extremely thin, his whole body in need of support. Visualize this young man, unable to even feed himself, being lifted from his wheelchair by his mother who holds him in her lap feeding him from a plate of food, they both share.

Each morning for 10 days, while I was staying at an ashram in India, I would see these two people at breakfast, the mother, about my own age, holding and feeding her son, about my own son's age, as if he were a baby. And always, the sweetest smile resting on both of their faces, as if they had the most wonderful secret. I was so drawn to these two that I would go particularly early to the Western canteen, in order to eat my breakfast near them. I sat at their table but several chairs away so as not to disturb them.

The love and devotion that these two people had for each other spilled out into the space around them and I soaked it up. It was a spiritual experience for me. It was as if I were bathing in the glow of the sun or a pure crystal lake. This young man was so physically deformed, his arms and legs were shriveled and he spoke in a slur impossible for me to understand from where I sat and yet there was something so beautiful about him, something about him that attracted me, something that charmed me. Each morning I would sit at their table as close as I could, to glimpse from the corner of my eye, this ritual between the mother and son. We never spoke or acknowledged each other. Neither the boy nor his mother ever looked in my direction.

On my last morning at the ashram, returning from the meditation mandir, I felt a strong pull over my right shoulder, as if I was being nudged to turn around. The most beautiful double rainbow had arched it-self right over the mandir. It seemed to begin at one side and end at the other. There were in fact two rainbows, one on top of the other and each rainbow was complete and separate, not really a double rainbow, which would have spun out from a common center of orange. These were sepa-rate and distinct. I had never before seen a display quite like this. About 50 yards behind me was the young man in his wheel chair with his mother. They noticed that I was looking at something behind them and turned to look. We must have been immersed in the rainbow for quite some time, for when I looked again there were a hundred or more people standing with their backs to me all absorbed in the miracle in the sky. As I was about to turn and continue on to my room to pack my bags, the young man turned his head toward me. Then his mother turned his wheelchair fully toward me and I became absorbed in the most beautiful smile I have ever seen from anybody, ever before or since. Even to this day I clearly recall the beauty of this young man. There was a pure crystal clear radiance of "spiritual beauty" emanating from him. It became quite clear to me that true "beauty" is a product of *ananda*, bliss and delight and this *ananda* was at the very essence of this young man. It is God-bright light, warm and comforting a true joyful expression of the Soul.

13. Questions and Answers

Question: How should we concentrate in practicing mantras?

Answer: Mantras are a language between levels of consciousness, so it is important to repeat them in such a way that one's consciousness both deepens and widens, like a seed which grows into a tree. In ordinary physical consciousness, our consciousness, even our identity is absorbed in the phenomena being experienced through the five senses. We are pre-occupied with what we are seeing, reading, hearing, feeling on the skin, etc. In ordinary dream consciousness, which includes daydreaming, our consciousness is also contracted and absorbed in memories, imaginations like anxiety, desire, judgments. To gain the benefit of mantra sadhana, therefore, one needs to concentrate on not only the sound or pronunciation of the mantra, but also on its meaning and what it is pointing to. The meaning may best be understood as a *bhava* or feeling, associated with such as ideas as love, surrender, strength, wisdom, abundance, radiance, peace.

The benefit will be even greater if one can remember the state of consciousness one felt when one was first initiated into the mantra. The mantra is essentially a vehicle of consciousness, and it reminds us of that state which we were in during the initiation. Mantra initiation is such a sacred event, and requires much preparation on the part of both the initiator and the one receiving initiation. It is rare that for example, we observe a day of silence, and intensive practice of Yoga, and chanting around a mantra yagna fire, as we did prior to the mantra initiation. So, remember that state of consciousness, with its love, purity, equanimity, the wide calm and energy which you cultivated before and during mantra initiation.

The seed syllables germinate during the mantra initiation. Later, as one practices them on one's own, they will grow in an expansive way like a plant, if when practicing them, one sets aside other preoccupations. One may do this during routine activities that do not require much concentration, like walking or riding in a car, and even driving the car if one is on a familiar route without much traffic. Such practice also helps us to weed out mental anxiety and trivial thinking, which ordinarily drains us of our mental energy.

If practiced with an aspiration for that to which the mantra corresponds, whether it be love, wisdom, strength, abundance, enlightenment, for example, one creates the ideal conditions in which such states come down from the mental plane and manifest, even magically in the material plane. As our life is largely the consequence of our past thoughts, words and actions, that is our karma, as we replace old habitual thoughts with the mantra, the old karma tendencies lose their force and dry up. Such an aspiration however, must not contain any impatience, hope or doubt. It must be filled with feelings of confidence in the efficacy of the power of the mantra, and surrender to the Will of the Divine. The highest aspiration, is simply "Not my will, but Thy will be done." Then whatever one recieves, will be in alignment with the Will of the Divine, and one will overcome the ego-based illusion of being "the doer."

When our minds are troubled by life's challenges, the practice of the mantras can be performed as a kind of balm, to soothe the anxiety, sadness or agitation in the mind. Even if the mind is competing with the mantra recitation, the latter will gradually wear down the mental chatter, leaving one in a peaceful state.

Mantras can be done prior to the practice of meditation as an aid to calming and concentrating the mind, and preparing it for meditation.

It is best to practice the mantra continuously during a given period, or for a predetermined number, in order to develop one's will power; however, if circumstances demand that you put your attention elsewhere, the mantra sadhana should be temporarily put aside, until one can return to it with full or near full attention.

Question: How to balance internal and external focus, in order to optimize both?

Answer: By "internal focus" you are most likely referring to the Witness state of consciousness. By "external focus," you are probably referring to concentration on the tasks at hand, or being attentive. Both states are to be valued, and have their time and place. What we seek in Yoga is not either or only one of these, but rather to purify our mind of the ego-sense, which causes us to feel that "I am the doer," Or "I am the body-mind-personality."

"Internal focus" is what most meditative or spiritual traditions encourage, and it provides a much needed balance to the ordinary materialistic and sensual based mentality which modern culture encourages. Particularly today, our culture encourages us to believe that the more things we can experience, the happier we will be. However, this encourages one to confuse happiness, which is always an internal experience with external things, persons or phenomena. Meditative and spiritual traditions begin by helping the beginner to slow down, simplify, and turn within, so as to find one's calm inner being, one's center, one's spirit or soul, which has the qualities of awareness, light, equanimity, transcendence, joy and peace.

There is a risk however, that the discovery of one's spiritual dimension may bring a denial of the other dimensions of one's life: the physical, emotional, mental and intellectual, particularly in those cultures or traditions which are *mayavadin*, that is, see the world as an objective illusion.

They often encourage a renunciation of the world. This is the predominant tradition in Asia, even today, as it was in the West until the time of the Renaissance. In our modern materialistic culture, however, only a few are tempted to go to such an extreme. The vast majority of meditators in the West use their practice as a means of relieving the stress of their daily lives, and at best as a means of cultivating the spiritual dimension, which has been normally neglected.

At some point, however, the spiritual dimension's inherent joy and well-being begins to overflow into one's daily life. One begins to feel a wide calm, even peace and acceptance as to how things are, even as one goes about the routine activities and the challenging experiences of ordinary life. However, everyone is still running on their old programs, or *samskaras,* and until these are sufficiently weakened, and replaced with more sattvic or wisdom based tendencies, such states of calm and peace can still be overwhelmed by the events of daily life.

Therefore, the question of how to balance the "internal focus" with the "external focus," is essentially answered by the prescription "to be calmly active and actively calm." Most of the techniques of Yoga have as their purpose the cultivation of this middle path, known as *sattva,* which is characterized by the qualities of balance, lightness, awareness, peace, calm, and intelligence. As our practice of Yoga deepens and widens, *sattva* grows even in our daily life. Because our human nature is so habitual, however, one must engage in Yogic sadhana regularly, patiently and persistently. One must also be well informed by a "road map" or classic text of Yoga, so as to be able to recognize the pitfalls, the obstacles and how to surmount them: "Disease, dullness, doubt, carelessness, laziness, sense indulgence, false perception, failure to reach firm ground, and instability." (Yoga Sutra I.30) Sadhana weakens *samskaras*, and enables us to act consciously, rather than to react habitually.

By cultivating presence, awareness comes, and when awareness comes, bliss comes as well. In such a state of being, consciousness and bliss, all actions can be performed without the distortion of the ego. One acts as an instrument, skilfully, without attachment to the results; one's joy is Self-evident, and independent of whether or not the action produces the results desired or expected.

In terms of·practice, cultivate the Witness state first during routine activities, like dishwashing, housecleaning, walking, eating, bathing, from the beginning to the end, continuously. As the Witness state becomes more stable, remember it during activities that require more concentration or attention: repairing something, shopping, listening to someone speak on the telephone; later when it is more firmly established, cultivate it while the mind is engaged in reading or other activities that require much concentration. Even then, part of the consciousness can remain as a Witness, in a state of "internal focus," while the rest of the consciousness is concentrating on the tasks or challenges at hand, i.e. "external focus." If most of your time is absorbed in challenging activities that require much "external focus" then find ways to simplify, so you can reserve more time for pastimes, which will enable you to cultivate "internal focus.".

Why is this important? It is what I like to refer to as "the game of consciousness." Every time you play it, that is, you practice being present and aware, that is the Witness, bliss appears. Guaranteed! And every time you forget to be the Witness, suffering appears. Automatically. You can easily test this. Awareness is the only game in life where you always win. In all the other games, you ultimately lose, because only Presence, Consciousness and Bliss are eternal and infinite. Everything else is limited by time or space, and is hence, temporary.

Question: In Advaita Vedanta, one focuses only on the Self. Why do we have other points of focus in Babaji's Kriya Yoga?

Answer: There are six major systems of philosophy in India, including the philosophy of non-dualism, "Advaita Vedanta," and Samkhya, upon which Yoga is based. The goal of Advaita Vedanta is to realize the Self, That which eternally is, in the spiritual plane. All else is held to be an objective illusion, if not simply a distraction. The philosophical system known as Saiva Siddhantha, or "final, perfect Truth of the knowers of Shiva" expresses what the Tamil Yoga Siddhas, the originators of Babaji's Kriya Yoga crystallized in the form of practical yogic techniques. In the Siddhantha the world is not considered to be an illusion, or *maya*. Rather, the mind may be subject to delusion, to due its fundamental ignorance, but this does not change the objective reality of the world. By understanding the world, including our own Nature, the Siddhas were able to realize their full potential in all five dimensions of existence: physical, vital, mental, intellectual and spiritual.

Saiva Siddhantha begins where Vedanta ends, so said one of the greatest modern exponents of the Siddha system, Yogi Ramaiah, under the inspiration of Satguru Babaji Nagaraj. Their teachings are known as "Tamil Kriya Yoga Siddhantham," and we belong to their tradition. After realizing One-ness of the spiritual plane of existence the Tamil Yoga Siddhas realized that the ultimate Truth was to be surrendered to on all levels, including the spiritual, intellectual, mental, vital and physical. They developed the Kriyas to permit mastery of human nature in all five bodies. When one has real-ized God on the spiritual plane, one may be called a "saint," or God knower; when realized on the intellectual plane, one may be called a "sage," one who can express truth extemporaneously in any field of knowledge with great intuitive insight; when one realizes God on the men-tal plane, one becomes a Siddha, one who possesses "siddhis," or yogic mi-raculous powers involving the subtle senses of sight, clairvoyance, of hear-ing, clairaudience, etc. When one surrenders the ego to the Divine con-sciousness even on the spiritual plane, the even greater *siddhis* manifest, which involve materialization and dematerialization, mind over matter, wish fulfilment, awareness of reality at the atomic and cosmic levels. In the case of a very few "Maha Siddhas" like Babaji and his gurus Agastyar and Bogar, even the consciousness of physical cells of the body surrender to the Divine consciousness, and so become as eternal as the Divine. Enlighten-ment in a diseased body cannot be considered to be perfection or siddhi, no matter how great the spiritual attainment.

In practical terms, to try to only concentrate on the most sublime part of our being, the Self, at the spiritual level, is certainly the most direct means, but very few persons have the steadiness or willpower to do so. Their lower nature is just too powerful. So, the Siddhas developed practical techniques or "kriyas" to help them to overcome the lower nature; Siddhas like Patan-jali developed a step by step process wherein one gradually develops the requisite purity, physical and mental calmness, concentration, sense with-drawal before reaching *samadhi*. Those who attempt to reach *samadhi* in the spiritual plane directly, unaided by such methods are usually over-whelmed by adverse reactions from the physical, vital, mental, and intel-lectual nature.

Also, by developing our ability to master the mind, vital and physical we can become a more complete instrument of the Divine in this world. Rather than seeking heaven or liberation from this world, the Siddhas like Babaji dedicated themselves to serving the evolution of all of its living in-habitants.

Question: How does Babaji's Kriya Yoga compare with the Kriya Yoga promoted by Yogananda and his successors?

Answer: Yogananda faced the daunting task of a pioneer trying to introduce yoga in a largely hostile environment, where there was a tremendous amount of ignorance, scepticism and even fear with regards to yoga in what was a fundamentalist Christian culture. For the first five years of his stay in America, from 1920 to 1925, while residing in Arlington, Massachusetts, just north of Cambridge, one of the most liberal places in America, he tried to teach yoga and Indian spirituality as he had learned it. Only a handful of persons responded. He felt that his mission called him to reach large numbers of persons in the West, so he cut his hair, stopped wearing ochre-colored cloth in public, except for special occasions, and transformed his vocabulary and theology from that of Hinduism to that of Christianity. He asked for $10,000 from his chief benefactor, Dr. Lewis, to go on a cross country lecture tour. It was during crossroads in his life Yogananda began simplifying the teaching of Kriya Yoga, by eliminating the postures, concentrating on only two simple meditations, the sound of "Om," and "Hong-Sau," and greatly simplifying the practice of Kriya Kundalini pranayama. "Va-Shee" became "Ah-eee," to avoid offending fundamentalist Christians who might feel that repeating the name "Shiva" would be blasphemous. In this way he could initiate in less than an hour a thousand people at a time sitting in an auditorium. In the second initiation, which was given only to a relatively small number of persons, a meditation on mantras with the chakras was given. Yogananda also promoted "self-energizing" exercises, which involved mostly static contraction of various groups of muscles. It was a unique variation of ancient techniques, but it enabled many Westerners to keep fit, without doing Hatha Yoga. During the 1920's and 1930's there were many theories about differences between the races, and it was commonly believed up until the 60's that Westerners could not practice the yoga asana (postures) because their bodies were ill suited to doing them.

Yogananda's great contribution, however, aside from getting many persons started on the path of yoga, was his metaphysical writings. Most of these have been published in book form. The correspondence course lessons, which are required reading prior to initiation by the SRF, are excerpts from these publications. They are a wonderful source of guidance in how to live one's life. He greatly emphasized the use of "affirmations," which like their more modern forms of "auto-hypnosis" and "neuro-linguistic programming," seeks to change deep-rooted subconscious attitudes.

Yogananda's personal spiritual orientation was towards the "Divine Mother," but he was wise enough not to emphasize it in our culture, where God is only a "He," and so he put at the center of his work a Christian theology and devotional practice. The services, which he organized were along the lines of a Protestant style church service, with hymns, prayers, songs focused on the person of Jesus, in particular. He called us to attain "Christ Consciousness," with apt interpretations from selected quotations from the New Testament Bible to support the marriage of Western Christianity and Eastern yoga. He did not even reveal the person of Babaji, the origin of Kriya Yoga and his mission until 1946, when the first edition of his "Autobiography of a Yogi" was published.

Finally, Yogananda remained faithful to the Western religious model by passing the mantle of his mission to an organization, the Self Realization Fellowship, declaring that there would be no further "gurus" in the SRF line, but that his correspondence course lessons would fulfil that role.

The SRF has become a zealous guardian of Yogananda's teaching. It has promoted them mostly through publications, a three year weekly correspondence course, and occasional forays into distant cities by SRF monks to give lectures and initiation ceremonies, which last about an hour. The SRF has also been a jealous guardian, having spent more than 10 million dollars in legal fees in recent years in trying to destroy its rival, the Ananda Church of Self-Realization, when they began publishing Yogananda's writing and pictures. The SRF now declares itself to be a religion, and admonishes its members to avoid reading from other spiritual traditions and to avoid following other spiritual teachers or teachings. It adheres strictly to Yogananda's teachings, so much so, that if a student raises a question which is not addressed in the SRF lessons; it is dismissed as being "unimportant."

All of our readers can compare the above with the five-fold path of "Babaji's Kriya Yoga," with its emphasis on yoga asanas, Kriya Kundalini pranayama, numerous dhyana kriyas, mantras and bhakti yoga. Babaji's Kriya Yoga is a complete and elaborate system of 144 Kriya or techniques, which encompass all five dimensions of human existence: the physical, vital, mental, intellectual and the spiritual. These require years of training in progressive stages.

Rather than choosing for its practitioners the Divine form, which they should worship, we encourage them to follow their own heart. Babaji's Kriya Yoga is the practical side of all world religions. It is not a religion, which involves a particular belief system. It is a scientific art, which requires practice and skill and its results can be scientifically replicated. It is not a belief system, requiring its members to avoid other belief systems. Its practitioners are encouraged to seek God and Self-realization from all sources. Yogananda himself learned Kriya Yoga from several different gurus, and was inspired by many more, as reported in his "Autobiography."

As in all Indian spiritual traditions, the flame is passed from one soul to another, not from an organization. In India, it is the sacred texts and the gurus who assure the passing of spiritual truths from one generation to another, and historically, this is done largely without formal organizations. In the West, religion is controlled by institutions, which are organizations which have usually put their own growth and survival ahead of the interests of their members. The Abrahamic religions are fear based, and their adherents often feel more comfortable with belonging to an organization or religion, which will save them from hell. In recent years however, under the influence of Eastern spirituality, adherence to "organized religion" in the West has waned significantly. More and more persons declare themselves to be "spiritual" rather than religious, and seek inspiration from many sources, without belonging to any particular organization.

In India, belief systems are considered to be constructions of the mind and only a starting point in one's spiritual quest. One's karma or personal efforts determines one's fate, although the effect of grace is also sought. It is probably fair to say that no one has ever become Self-realized because they adhered to an organization, or believed in some religious or philosophical belief system. It would be as far fetched as claiming, as one contemporary Indian guru does, that simply because of his father's and grandfather's spiritual realization, that he is "dynastically" Self realized!

Books and writings can only take us so far, to the limits of the intellect. Words and books tend to divide us. That is why Babaji's Kriya Yoga puts emphasis on a five fold path of practice of "yogic sadhana," all those practices, which remind one of the Presence, of Self Realization. It is a balanced path that seeks the transformation of the individual, not just spiritually, but physically, vitally, mentally and intellectually as well.

Babaji is at the center of our tradition. The Guru *tattva*, or principle by which truth, unconditional love, and wisdom is revealed, manifests through him and the Kriya Yoga which he developed as a synthesis of ancient esoteric teachings. He is its living source and fountainhead, who by example and inspiration, guides us. He is the only guru of our tradition. While the SRF considers Babaji to be one of its gurus, there is little mention of Babaji in the SRF literature; he is considered to be a historical personality, no longer on the physical plane, remote, inaccessible, with nothing to do with its direction.

The SRF is a Christian church with membership requirements. Furthermore it has declared itself to be a religion. It interprets "Christ" as a state of consciousness to be attained through the practice of Kriya Yoga. It is in this way that one is "saved" according to SRF theology. It conducts religious services like any Christian church, and its teachings are disseminated through SRF ministers. It prohibits its members from seeking guidance from any other spiritual teacher or organization.

Initiates of Babaji's Kriya Yoga are free to seek inspiration from all sources. There is no organization to which one becomes a member. The relationship between the initiate and Babaji is entirely personal. Babaji's Kriya Yoga is disseminated through a network of initiates who volunteer their services. Some are trained as instructors in Babaji's Kriya Hatha Yoga and basic techniques of breathing, meditation and yogic philosophy. Advanced and qualified students may be invited to become members of a small lay order of teachers, Babaji's Kriya Yoga Order of Acharyas. After fulfilling rigorous conditions, they are authorized to initiate others into Babaji's Kriya Yoga Kriya Kundalini Pranayam and meditation techniques, and subsequently some also initiate others into mantras and all 144 kriyas in the system.

Questions are encouraged in Babaji's Kriya Yoga, not as a means of cultivating doubts, but as a constructive way to convert doubts into steps towards Self-realization. Babaji's Kriya Yoga is a living, oral, tradition, growing in the hearts and experience of its practitioners. It is not confined between book covers, or the stories of its leaders, or the walls of an institution.

Babaji's Kriya Yoga is inspired by the teachings of the 18 Tamil Yoga Siddhas, such as is found in "Thirumandiram," as well as the "Sanatana Dharma," "the eternal religion" of India. The Siddhas, however, emphasized that God was not to be found only in temples or elaborate ceremonies, but with our hearts, by stripping away the veils of ignorance, desire and egoism. May everyone learn Babaji's Kriya Yoga and reach God realization, enjoying eternal peace and joy in all five planes of existence.

For information on Babaji's Kriya Yoga please contact:

Babaji's Kriya Yoga and Publications, Inc.
196 Mountain Road · P.O. Box 90
Eastman, Quebec · Canada J0E 1P0
Tel: +1(888) 252-9642 · +1(450) 297-0258 · Fax: +1(450) 297-3957
www.babajiskriyayoga.net · info@babajiskriyayoga.net

The Grace of Babaji's Kriya Yoga

A Course of Lessons

An Invitation from Babaji's Kriya Yoga and Publications, Inc.

Two years of Self- Exploration & Discovery

"To hope for a change in human life without a change in human nature is an irrational & un-spiritual proposition; it is to ask for something unnatural & unreal, an impossible miracle." Sri Aurobindo

In our pursuit of our Divine Self we must seek for change in our human nature. But rather than trying to change our nature, we more often merely attempt to reconcile our habits of desire, aversion and fear. So dark elements along with light continue to seek manifestation and arise in the context of our life.

The Grace Course provokes us to delve into our desires, aversions and fears in order to reveal to us our truth and falseness.

As ingrained habits and instincts are probed, weaknesses will be amplified. This process is personal and profound and real work.

Have You Sincerely and Genuinely Considered:

- How far can discipline and personal effort get you?
- What is Grace and is it absolutely necessary for Self-Knowledge?
- Is your Ego really so bad?
- Must I love everyone, or just do my duty?
- How can I keep love from diminishing into attachment or dissolving into anger or indifference?
- Why is life so full of desire, aversion and fear?
- Is there ever a need for fear?
- How can I learn to use my willpower effectively to overcome my resistances?
- Is there a Higher Will for my life, and if so, how can I learn to connect with it?
- Is what you can "see," even in meditation, ever the true Self?

The entire course consists of 24 monthly lessons. Each lesson is about 15 pages. You may subscribe one year at a time: $125 per year

To subscribe to this course, contact us at: **Babaji's Kriya Yoga Publications**

196 Mountain Road · PO Box 90 · Eastman · QC · J0E 1P0 Canada · **www.babajiskriyayoga.net**

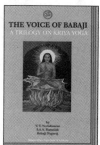
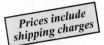
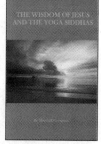
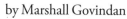
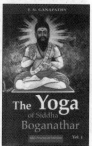

Other titles available from Kriya Yoga Publications, Inc.:

KRIYA YOGA SUTRAS OF PATANJALI AND THE SIDDHAS

by Marshall Govindan

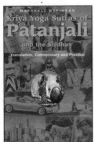

This translation is both easy to understand and precise. The commentary reveals for the first time the closeness of Patanjali to the Tamil Siddha philosophical tradition. A unique commentary which provides for each verse "practices" or Kriyas useful for the Kriya Yoga initiate and non-initiate alike. **"Indispensable for students of Kriya Yoga... a valuable addition to the study of Yoga in general and the Yoga-Sutra in particular. I can wholeheartedly recommend it."** From the foreword by Georg Feuerstein, Ph D. **"An excellent and easily readable commentary"** - David Frawley. **"A significant contribution to the sadhana of every serious yoga student"** - Yoga Journal. 220 pages, Sanskrit transliteration, indexes of Sanskrit and English terms, index of Kriyas indicated in the verses. ISBN 978-1-895383-12-6. Canada: CAD$34.37, USA: US$27.00, Asia & Europe: US$52.50

BABAJI'S KRIYA HATHA YOGA SELF-REALIZATION THROUGH ACTION WITH AWARENESS

DVD

With Marshall Govindan & Durga Ahlund

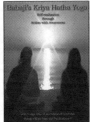

Learn the 18 postures developed by Babaji Nagaraj and become the Seer, not the Seen! Become aware of what is aware! Bliss arises! This unique, beautiful, 2 hour video provides careful detailed instructions in not only the technical performance of each posture, but also in the higher states of consciousness which they awaken. Make your practice of yoga deeply meditative. Taught in progressive stages with preparatory variations making them accessible to the beginner and challenging for the experienced student of Yoga.**"Earnest, unique and inspiring"** - Yoga Journal. ISBN 978-1-895383-18-8. Canada: CAD$24.94, Quebec: CN$26.51, USA: US$23.94, Asia & Europe: US$27.95

THE YOGA OF THE 18 SIDDHAS: AN ANTHOLOGY

Edited by T.N. Ganapathy

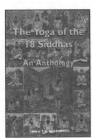

The Yoga of the Eighteen Siddhas: An Anthology includes a biography, an English translation and commentary of selected poems for each of the 18 Siddhas. It contains not only revolutionary statements of those great men and women who have reached the furthest heights of human potential, but also serves as a roadmap for the rest of us to follow. The Siddhas who represent the best of what we can all aspire to become have given us illuminated writings, so filled with the light of God realization that they can have an impact on our heart and mind, just by studying them. This book takes us along a path of Jnana Yoga. 642 pages. ISBN 978-1-895383-24-9. Canada: CAD$40.14, USA: US$32.50, Asia & Europe: US$74.50

To order our publications or tapes:

Call toll free: 1-888-252-9642 or (450) 297-0258, Fax: (450) 297-3957, E-mail: info@babajiskriyayoga.net

You may have your order charged to a VISA/MasterCard/AmericanExpress or send a cheque or International money order to:

Kriya Yoga Publications, P.O. Box 90, Eastman, Quebec, Canada, J0E 1P0

All prices include postal shipping charges and taxes.
or place your order securely via our E-commerce at www.babajiskriyayoga.net

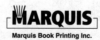

Marquis Book Printing Inc.

Québec, Canada
2008

  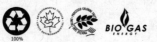 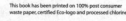

This book has been printed on 100% post consumer
waste paper, certified Eco-logo and processed chlorine free.

100%